Women's Edge
HEALTH ENHANCEMENT GUIDE™

Growing Younger

Breakthrough Age-Defying Secrets

By Julia VanTine, Bridget Doherty, and the Editors of

RODALE

Notice

This book is intended as a reference volume only, not as a medical manual. The information given here is designed to help you make informed decisions about your health. It is not intended as a substitute for any treatment that may have been prescribed by your doctor. If you suspect that you have a medical problem, we urge you to seek competent medical help.

Library of Congress Cataloging-in-Publication Data

VanTine, Julia.
    Growing younger : breakthrough age-defying secrets / by Julia VanTine,
Bridget Doherty, and the editors of Prevention Health Books
for Women.
      p. cm. — (Women's edge health enhancement guide)
    Includes index.
    ISBN 1–57954–120–8 hardcover
    1. Rejuvenation. 2. Longevity. 3. Youthfulness. 4. Women—Care
and hygiene. I. Doherty, Bridget. II. Prevention Health Books.
III. Title. IV. Series.
RA776.75.V36 1999
613'.04244—dc21   99–39654

Distributed to the book trade by St. Martin's Press

6 8 10 9 7   hardcover

Visit us on the Web at www.rodalebooks.com, or call us toll-free at (800) 848-4735.

RODALE
WE **INSPIRE** AND **ENABLE** PEOPLE TO IMPROVE
THEIR LIVES AND THE WORLD AROUND THEM

Prevention Health Books for Women Board of Advisors

Seeking Cinderella

When I was growing up, most of the older women I knew either hated to reveal their age or, worse, lied about it. (My mother was always 39.) I could never understand why they did that. Until now.

I dreaded my last birthday so much that I spent the entire year leading up to it repeating that two-syllable number aloud just to get used to the sound of it. Clever strategy. Didn't work.

So it was with great personal interest that I sent the writers and editor of this volume of the Women's Edge health series out to uncover the secrets that would help me hang on to fading youth.

Wow! Did they ever turn my head around. Aging ain't what it used to be!

Forget everything you ever heard about getting older. We baby boomers (okay, so now you know I'm somewhere between the ages of 36 and 54) are redefining what aging in America is all about. It's not about putting in time until retirement, forgetting where we put the car keys, or accepting the inevitable middle-age spread and sore joints. It's about starting second careers, boosting our mind power, loving our bodies, and defying the diseases that used to make women old before their time.

Everything you need to know about stopping the clock can be found in this volume: the foods that will keep you slim, glowing, and disease-free; the makeup and clothes that will turn heads; the supplements that will boost metabolism and rev your energy level; the attitude that will renew your spirit.

In fact, you'll learn that chronological years have hardly anything at all to do with aging. How old you *really* are is purely a state of mind, fostered by how good you feel about yourself and the state of your health.

After reading this book, I don't mind at all telling you how old I feel. Would you believe 39?

Anne Alexander
Editor-in-Chief, *Prevention* Magazine

Contents

PART ONE

The
Anti-Aging
Arsenal

The Anti-Aging Generation

At age 62, Deane Feetham wins triathlons. That's right. Her apartment in Anchorage, Alaska, is cluttered with trophies and ribbons from victories in those all-day, grueling sweatfests of running, biking, and swimming, even though she was in her midforties before her running shoes or bicycle wheels ever got a workout.

Of course, that's only what she does in her *spare* time. Feetham also holds down a day job selling supplies for a printing company. She has two grown daughters who adore her, a wide circle of friends, and volunteer work she loves. (She's a facilitator for an area breast-cancer survival group.) And she's studying exercise science at the University of Alaska with the eventual goal of becoming a physical trainer for older women. She has a fire in her belly and a light in her eye.

Aging, Baby-Boomer Style

Most of us probably don't share Feetham's passion for running. But it's likely that we share at least one thing with her: a conviction that growing older doesn't mean growing *old*.

"The idea of getting old just kind of doesn't exist for me," she says.

She isn't the only one who feels this way.

Our entire generation of baby boomers—the approximately 39 million women born between 1946 and 1964—have a radically different idea of what *old* is, and we ain't it. Just as we once redefined this country's social and political landscape, we're now redefining youthfulness as 'positive aging,' meaning extended physical health and vitality combined with a fresh and lively mental attitude.

But it isn't just our idea of aging that's changed. We're actually living longer . . . and better.

"This generation of women is living much longer past menopause than those of previous generations," says Vivian Pinn, M.D., associate director for research on women's health and director of the Office of Research on Women's Health at the National Institutes of Health in Bethesda, Maryland. "Over the past 10-plus years, we have made tremendous strides. Women now enjoy unprecedented opportunities for preserving and improving their health."

Why We Can Live Longer and Better

From the civil-rights movement to the Vietnam War, our generation experienced a unique time in American history. We were also fortunate enough to be born in an era of constant medical discoveries and advances.

In this century alone, a woman's life expectancy has increased by 31 years (a man's, by 26 years). The average woman now lives to be 79, the average man, 72. Moreover, the rate of disabilities among older people has dropped dramatically, most likely because of medical breakthroughs, better nutrition, and a decline in cigarette smoking.

We also stand to benefit from the recent explosion of research into women's health, particularly the health of women at midlife and beyond.

The Women's Health Initiative (WHI), a long-term national health study of heart disease, cancer, stroke, and osteoporosis in some 160,000 women ages 50 and over, is one of the largest prevention studies of its kind. It is examining the effect of hormone-replacement therapy (HRT) on the prevention of heart disease, osteoporosis, and breast and endometrial cancers; the effect of a healthy diet on the prevention of heart disease and breast and col-

THE GIFTS OF AGING

Maybe we don't have the body we had when we were 20, but growing older isn't without its perks, says Sue Patton Thoele, a licensed psychotherapist in Boulder, Colorado, and author of *Freedoms after 50*. Below is her top-10 list of aging's more subtle gifts.

We can act "disgracefully." "To me, that's laughing uproariously in public, throwing your arms around a dear friend you haven't seen in a long time, using some spicy words to make your point. We're free to ignite the fiery part of ourselves."

We can take care of ourselves—and we know it. "For me, one of the benefits of aging is a deep, hard-earned trust in my ability to regain my equilibrium when I'm knocked off-kilter."

We can just say no. Period. "Being able to say that wonderfully assertive word without guilt, explanation, or remorse is to break free from the prison of obligation. At our age, we've certainly earned the privilege."

We have more time to let our creative juices flow. "Most of us have more leisure time as we get older, so we can develop our creativity more fully. And since we don't have to prove ourselves, we're more inclined to try anything."

Sex becomes more spiritual. "There's a depth of feeling between you and your mate that makes sex less about performance and more about tenderness and sharing."

We don't have to cook if we don't want to. "There are many times now when I grant myself the freedom to assert my noncooking credo of 'Forage, take out, or take me out.'"

We can snooze when we choose. "Pets are admirable nappers, able to doze off whenever the mood strikes. We now have the time to follow their example."

We can can the guilt. "There's a saying, 'Show me a woman without guilt, and I'll show you a man.' It's time that we kiss guilt goodbye."

We learn to accept things as they are. "One of the joys of maturity is realizing that it's perfectly all right to give up trying to control everything and accept what is. What a blessed relief."

Our "wisdom gland" kicks in. "With our wealth of experience, we gain perspective—a much deeper understanding of what's *really* important in our lives."

LIFE EXTENDER
Eat Candy, Live Longer

A longer life is often a sweeter life, according to research conducted at the Harvard School of Public Health.

Researchers tracked the health and lifestyle habits of 7,841 men who entered Harvard between 1916 and 1950. They found that those who occasionally splurged on a sweet treat lived almost a year longer than men who did not eat any candy.

As in all things, however, moderation is key. Candy lovers who ate from one to three sweets a month lived longer than those who gobbled them three or more times a week. "While our research included only men, it is likely that the same biologic processes operate in women," says study leader I-Min Lee, M.D., assistant professor of epidemiology at the Harvard School of Public Health. "So the findings should apply to women as well."

orectal cancers; and the effect of calcium and vitamin D supplementation on the prevention of osteoporosis and colorectal cancer.

The emerging field of gender-based biology, which examines the biological and physiological differences between women and men, has already made discoveries with potential long-term health implications. According to the Society for Women's Health Research, it is now known that women who smoke are 20 to 70 percent more likely to develop lung cancer than men who smoke the same number of cigarettes. They are more likely than men to suffer a second heart attack within a year of their first. And they can metabolize medications differently from the way men do.

We have access to a mind-boggling amount of health information, says Florence Haseltine, M.D., founder of the Society for Women's Health Research, now director of the Center for Population Research at the National Institutes of Health in Washington, D.C. From morning news shows to the Internet, never has there been so much coverage of women's health. With more information, we're in a better position to make informed health-related decisions that can affect the length and quality of our lives.

Finally, we boomer women are discriminating—and vocal—healthcare consumers. In the 1970s, we took on the medical establishment over reproductive health issues such as access to birth control and abortion. As we enter menopause, we're still challenging conventional medical wisdom. In fact, our generation of women has been credited for fueling interest in alternative medicine in this country. One study found that 4 of every 10 Americans used alternative therapies in 1997, including more than half of people between 30 and 50 years old.

Our New Health Strategy: Defense

When our moms were young, people who ate more vegetables than meat, exercised regularly, and took vitamins were considered, well, a bit strange. The all-American way to age was to accept that you would get sick—"old" people always did—and that a kindly, wise Marcus Welby type would make all of your medical decisions for you.

Not anymore. Our generation has a new focus: preventing age-related diseases before they strike us. "Women are saying, 'Okay, we're living longer. We want to know more about how to prevent illnesses that can keep us from enjoying these longer years of life,'" says Dr. Pinn.

It's long been known that a healthy diet and regular exercise help prevent many of the illnesses associated with aging, such as cancer, diabetes, and especially cardiovascular disease, which kills more women than all forms of cancer combined.

What's new, however, is the growing evidence that antioxidants and plant chemicals (phytochemicals) in fruits and vegetables may also stave off age-related diseases, including diabetes, macular degeneration, and breast cancer. Found in our bodies as well as in fruits and vegetables, antioxidants neutralize free radicals, which are "crippled" oxygen molecules that steal electrons from our healthy cells and cause aging and illness.

For example, soy foods, such as tofu and soy milk, are rich in phytoestrogens, natural substances in soybeans that show great promise in preventing breast cancer, osteoporosis, and menopausal hot flashes. And one Swedish study of women over 50 found that women who consumed daily the amount of beta-carotene found in half a carrot had up to 68 percent less risk for breast cancer than women who ate the least.

As for exercise, "it's the best anti-aging medicine in the world," says Andrea Z. LaCroix, Ph.D., professor of epidemiology at Group Health Cooperative of Puget Sound in Seattle. Lifelong exercise may add as much as 7 years to our life span. Studies suggest that regular exercise may boost our bodies' levels of antioxidants, preventing the free-radical damage that gums up our works.

Free at Last

One of the most important "breakthroughs" in women's health is our generation's radically different take on menopause. "The women's health movement has brought menopause out of the closet," says Dr. Pinn. "Women don't fear it anymore. They understand that it's a natural part of our maturing and that it marks the beginning of the rest of our lives."

One poll of 750 women between the ages of 45 and 60 found that 52 percent viewed menopause as a new and fulfilling stage of life, 60 percent did not feel that menopause made them less attractive, and 80 percent said that they were actually relieved that their periods had stopped.

In our mothers' day, women may have whispered about "the change" behind closed doors, but now we form menopause support groups and actively seek information on menopause and hormone-replacement therapy. We play a far more active role in our midlife health care than our mothers did. "There's a well-educated group of women who visit their doctors with a checklist of things they want information about, particularly HRT," says Ruth C. Fretts, M.D., assistant professor of obstetrics, gynecology, and reproductive biology at Harvard Medical School.

We're Hot—and We Don't Mean Hot Flashes

Not all of us went in for the free-love, if-it-feels-good-do-it attitude toward sex that began in the late 1960s. But many of us maintain a healthy interest in sex. In fact, in a large national study, women in their forties and fifties reported more orgasms than women in their early twenties.

In part, this increased sexual satisfaction has to do with more leisure time. "As we get older, there's less hurry-hurry and rush-rush. That attitude translates beautifully into the sexual arena," says Sue Patton Thoele, a licensed psy-

WOMEN ASK WHY

Why do women live longer than men?

There is a multitude of possible explanations. But the available evidence suggests that biological, behavioral, social, and psychological differences between men and women all play a part. The three biggies seem to be related to behavior, cardiovascular disease risk, and chromosomes.

More men tend to die of factors caused by reckless behavior or violence, whatever their age. In men ages 55 to 64, for example, behavior-related fatalities—car accidents, falls, drownings, homicides, suicides—are among the most common causes of death and are much higher in men than in women.

Cardiovascular disease hits men earlier than it does women. Smoking is a huge risk factor in heart disease, and men still smoke more than women. A man's risk of heart disease skyrockets beginning in his forties. A woman's risk doesn't rise until she enters menopause. Sex hormones may play a role here. It's known that the male sex hormone testosterone raises levels of artery-clogging low-density lipoprotein (LDL) cholesterol and decreases levels of beneficial high-density lipoprotein (HDL) cholesterol. Estrogen, the primary female sex hormone, lowers LDL and increases HDL.

The fact that women have two X chromosomes, while men have only one, may also explain our longevity edge. Recent research suggests that the X chromosome may directly determine life span. One of a woman's two X chromosomes is inactivated early in life. But the second appears to kick in as she grows older, and so it compensates for lost or damaged genes on the first X. So from a genetic standpoint, women may just start out healthier.

Continuing research into the causes for the longevity gap will undoubtedly find clues to how both men and women can live longer, healthier lives.

Expert consulted
Ruth C. Fretts, M.D.
Assistant professor of obstetrics, gynecology,
and reproductive biology
Harvard Medical School

chotherapist in Boulder, Colorado, and author of *Freedoms after 50*. It doesn't hurt that the kids are out of the house and that we don't have to worry about unplanned pregnancy, she adds.

Because we know more about our bodies than our mothers did, we also have a better understanding of how to cope with the natural physical changes that can affect our sexuality. Vaginal dryness, for example, is easily remedied with lubricants. And while we take longer to become physically aroused—about 5 minutes, compared to premenopausal women's 10 to 15 seconds—even this has its benefits. Our partners take longer to become aroused, too. And didn't we always want a guy to take his time?

It's Our Turn Now

Few of us burned our bras in the 1970s, but to a large extent, that first wave of feminism gained us freedoms and opportunities that are helping to keep us young.

In attitude, that is.

Studies of older women find that, to many, midlife and beyond means more choices, more opportunities, more freedom—perks in short supply during our younger days. Instead of hitting the recliner, we're returning to school or to work, advancing in our careers, finding new interests, and discovering or rediscovering our talents.

"My research strongly supports the view that women are happier and more fulfilled as they age. Many feel that it's the best time in their lives," says Mary Guindon, Ph.D., associate professor of counseling in the department of graduate education at Rider University in Lawrenceville, New Jersey.

Released from the obligations of home and family, midlife women have incredible opportunities to develop themselves in any way they choose, says Dr. Guindon. Many women choose to go back to school.

Education is one predictor of successful aging. A study conducted at the California Public Health Foundation in Berkeley found that people with 12 years or more of education were healthier in their later years than those who had less schooling.

Many of us discover or rediscover our creative talents, which encompass everything from cooking to gardening to the arts. Others bring their creativity to volunteerism, another activity that research suggests increases our happiness and improves our health.

"One of my friends tapped her creativity by devising a plan to get food and supplies to an Indian reservation about 10 hours from where we live," says Thoele. "Last year, this woman was saying, 'I know I'm here for a reason. I just don't know what it is.' Now she does—and she's on fire."

There comes a point where women come into their own, says Dr. Guindon. "One 52-year-old woman from my study said, 'I used to think that 50 or 60 was old. But I'm energized. We're alive. We're out there. We need to plan for a long future because we're going to be out there for a very long time.'"

Grazing in the Garden of Youth

Pablo Picasso once said, "It takes a long time to become young." He could easily have added, "And a lot of food."

Yes, food.

There's no longer the slightest doubt that eating the right foods is one of the keys, if not *the* key, to preventing heart disease, cancer, and other age-related diseases. But now there's scientific evidence that a healthy diet can actually delay—or in some cases, even reverse—the aging process itself. Pretty cool, don't you think?

The right diet can encourage our bodies to produce "youth hormones" that control the ebb and flow of our bodies' anti-aging mechanisms, says Vincent C. Giampapa, M.D., president of the American Board of Anti-Aging Medicine and president of Longevity Institute International, a company based in Montclair, New Jersey, that provides personalized anti-aging programs through member physicians. The result: increased energy; stronger immunity; improvements in memory, vision, and hearing; more muscle; and denser bone.

Eating right can also help our cells repair and replace themselves more quickly, transport energy, and get rid of waste and toxins more efficiently. Just as important, diet can help protect our DNA, the genetic blueprint that tells our bodies' 50 to 60 trillion cells how to do their jobs.

Take a Bite Out of Aging

According to Dr. Giampapa, the goal of a "longevity diet" is to return our bodies to their youthful efficiency, which it can do in three ways.

Boost our youth hormones. The most important hormones for keeping us young are human growth hormone (hGH), which is released by the pituitary gland and converted in the liver to another anti-aging hormone called insulin growth factor (IGF-1), and dehydroepiandrosterone (DHEA), which is produced by the adrenal glands.

Starting in our twenties, our bodies slow down production of these hormones by about 10 percent every decade. By age 65, we are making only 15 to 20 percent of the hGH and 10 to 20 percent of the DHEA that we did when we were in our twenties.

With fewer youth hormones around, says Dr. Giampapa, chemical messages don't come and go as efficiently, which reduces the ability of our cells and organs to maintain and repair themselves. We experience loss of muscle and bone density, lowered immunity, and more illnesses, including diabetes and cancer.

Situation hopeless? Not quite.

"Increasing the body's production of these hormones can slow the aging process significantly," says Dr. Giampapa. "And it can be done primarily through diet."

Stem free-radical damage. Our cells use oxygen to produce energy. In the process, they generate free radicals—unstable oxygen molecules that damage cells and DNA. Free radicals are also produced by pollution, by the pesticides in our food supply, and by a diet high in chemical additives, refined starches and sugars, artery-clogging saturated fat found in meat, whole-milk dairy products, tropical oils, and foods like cookies and crackers that contain hydrogenated or partially hydrogenated oils.

Our bodies are good at fending off free radicals when we're young. But as we grow older, we start to lose some of that fight as the damage caused by years of exposure starts to take its toll. We begin to need help from antioxidant nutrients such as vitamins C and E, the minerals zinc and selenium, and the plant chemicals (phytochemicals) in many fruits and vegetables, which

LIFE EXTENDER
The Magic Mushroom

The Roman emperor Nero called mushrooms the food of the immortal gods. For thousands of years, healers in China and Japan have prized one particular variety, the maitake (pronounced "my-TAH-key"), believing it held the secret to longevity and immortality.

Is there truth in any of this?

According to modern science, there just may be. Research suggests that the succulent maitake may extend our lives by preventing or treating several age-related diseases.

Maitake D-fraction, an extract of the mushroom developed by Japanese researchers, seems to turn on certain cells in our immune systems (T cells), which then may help to fight cancer cells. Investigators have found evidence that maitake D-fraction may help prevent tumor growth, keep cancer from spreading from one part of the body to another, and prevent normal cells from mutating into cancer cells.

Maitake also contains compounds known as ES- and X-fractions, which, according to recent studies at Georgetown University, may help to lower levels of sugar and fats in the blood. In one Japanese laboratory study, maitake-enriched food significantly lowered levels of blood glucose and triglycerides after 8 weeks.

To get the most out of maitake, consume the D-fraction (available in capsules and tinctures), which is the most potent and active form, says Shari Lieberman, Ph.D., a nutrition scientist and exercise physiologist in New York City. Maitake is also sold in a tea. The various forms of maitake are available in gourmet markets and health food stores. Whole maitakes are considered to be the tastiest of the medicinal mushrooms.

Maitake D-fraction dissolves in hot water. If you steam or boil maitakes in their whole mushroom form, Dr. Lieberman suggests that you either consume the liquid in which they have been cooked or use it in soups, stews, or sauces. Also, don't stir-fry maitakes. The compounds responsible for lowering high blood sugar and high blood pressure levels will dissolve in the cooking oil.

join forces with our bodies' internal defense systems.

Replenish our "cellular soup." Each of our cells contains a substance called cytoplasm, which is made up of fluid, nutrients, and other materials that help make energy and fight free-radical damage, says Israel Kogan, M.D., director of the Anti-Aging Medical Center in Washington, D.C.

The typical American diet is loaded with chemical additives, pesticides and fertilizers, and other toxic substances, all of which encourage the formation of free radicals, says Dr. Kogan. When our diets are free of these toxins, we protect our cells from free-radical damage, give our cytoplasm the nutrients it needs, and help our cells to function at their peak.

A "clean" diet also helps return our bodies to the right level of acidity (pH), which is tremendously important in building up our cellular soup, says Dr. Giampapa. That's because our bodies make hormones, repair cells, and generally work most effectively at a neutral pH.

Check the Index

So how do we boost—or even hang on to—our youth hormones? One way is to skip the cherry-cheese Danish and enjoy the cherries straight. That's good advice for all the obvious reasons, but for a not-so-obvious one as well: Sugary pastries like that cherry-cheese Danish have what is known as a high glycemic index. The glycemic index measures how quickly a food raises our blood sugar levels after we eat it and how quickly our levels return to normal.

REAL-LIFE SCENARIO
A Vegetarian Who's Doing It All Wrong

Cheryl, a 42-year-old homemaker, had known for a long time that fast food, coffee, and playing supermom didn't exactly add up to a healthy lifestyle. But something she saw in the mirror one morning jolted her. Her skin and her eyes looked sallow and lifeless, which reflected exactly the way she felt: old. She made an instant decision to turn her life around. She knew where to start: cut out fatty foods and start an exercise program. Never one to do anything halfway, she became a vegetarian and began filling her plate with carbohydrates, such as macaroni and potatoes, to "boost her energy." She also started a vigorous weight-lifting program. But now, after weeks and weeks on her do-it-yourself rejuvenating program, she feels and looks more haggard than ever. And to make matters worse, she seems to have gained weight. What should she do?

While it may come as a surprise to Cheryl that she's feeling haggard and gaining weight, there may be two not-so-surprising culprits here: an unbalanced diet and, perhaps, a too-vigorous weight-training program.

First, Cheryl's diet. Vegetarian eating isn't automatically healthy eating. And, like many new vegetarians, Cheryl isn't consuming a balanced diet. While she may love macaroni, potatoes, and other starchy foods, they alone can't give her body the nutrients it needs to stay healthy, and they may even cause her to gain weight.

If Cheryl really wants to boost her energy—and improve her health—she needs to eat a wide variety of plant-based foods, including whole grains, legumes, and fresh fruits and vegetables. Legumes and whole grains should be the centerpiece of her diet. If Cheryl is a vegetarian who also eats dairy products (a lacto-vegetarian), she should choose low-fat milk and yogurt over their whole-fat counterparts.

Following these basic guidelines, Cheryl might breakfast on

Foods with a low glycemic index, like cherries, along with most fruits and vegetables and whole grains, encourage youthful levels of hGH and IGF-1, according to Dr. Giampapa.

a bowl of whole-grain cereal or oatmeal, topped with a sliced banana and a small amount of fat-free or soy milk. For lunch, she might opt for a vegetarian burger on a whole-grain bun with lettuce, tomato, and mustard or a bowl of hearty lentil soup with a slice of whole-grain bread. Dinner might be stir-fried vegetables over whole-grain brown rice or pasta.

Between meals, she might snack on fresh fruit, a piece of whole-grain bread spread with almond butter, or a cup of plain, low-fat yogurt with fresh fruit.

Consuming a wide variety of plant foods will also ensure that Cheryl gets adequate amounts of protein. Dried beans, such as chickpeas and black beans, are an excellent source of plant protein, as are grains, nuts, and seeds. If she's not crazy about seeds and grains, she can also get protein from more everyday foods, such as potatoes and broccoli.

Finally, Cheryl should consider taking a high-potency multivitamin/mineral supplement. It will be her "insurance" against missing out on essential vitamins and minerals.

Cheryl's weight gain is most likely caused by a combination of her vigorous weight-training program and her high-carbohydrate diet. Actually, a small weight gain from weight training is normal: Muscle weighs more than fat; so if she's putting on muscle, the needle on the scale will naturally go up. But again, her diet may be causing her to gain fat along with the muscle.

To lose the fat while keeping the muscle, Cheryl should watch her intake of sweets and other high-fat foods, even if they come from plant sources. She should also consider adding aerobic exercise to her program, which will burn calories and help her shed excess weight.

Expert consulted
Michael Janson, M.D.
President
American College for Advancement in Medicine
Barnstable, Massachusetts

They travel slowly through our digestive systems, so sugar enters our bloodstreams a little at a time, says Shari Lieberman, Ph.D., a nutrition scientist and exercise physiologist in New York City. This slow, steady rise in blood sugar promotes a stable release of insulin, the hormone that moves energy (glucose) from our blood to our cells.

When our insulin levels stay steady, our bodies produce less cortisol, often called the stress hormone, says Dr. Giampapa. That's good. Low cortisol levels encourage our bodies to produce DHEA as well as the hormones made from it.

By contrast, we digest high-glycemic foods, such as cornflakes, rice cakes, white potatoes, and white rice, more quickly. As a result, our blood sugar rises rapidly, triggering a flood of cortisol. High insulin and cortisol levels reduce our output of DHEA and the hormones made from it.

We can discourage these youth-stealing spikes in insulin and cortisol by eating mostly foods with a low to medium glycemic index, says Dr. Giampapa.

Aim Low

As you may have guessed by now, low-glycemic foods tend to be high in fiber and complex carbohydrates, while high-glycemic foods contain virtually none. Here's how to make your diet more "complex."

Eat heavyweight bread. Buy whole-grain bread that contains at least 3 grams of dietary fiber per slice, says Dr. Lieberman. It will have a much lower glycemic index than white bread or even low-calorie whole-wheat bread.

Rule of thumb: The heavier the loaf, the better. "The bread I eat? You can eat it or use it as a paperweight," says Dr. Lieberman. (While

LIFE EXTENDER

Eat Less, Live Longer

There's growing evidence that we may be able to extend our lives simply by eating less.

Studies of mice and rats have demonstrated that both live 30 percent longer when they consume 30 percent fewer calories. More recent laboratory studies conducted at Johns Hopkins University show that consuming a low-calorie, low-fat diet helps maintain higher levels of dehydroepiandrosterone (DHEA), a "youth hormone" produced by our bodies.

Experts aren't sure why eating less seems to slow aging. But a growing body of evidence suggests that reducing calories also reduces the body's production of age-accelerating free radicals.

dense bread contains more calories, it also fills you up, leaving you more satisfied.)

Pass on the lightweight cereal. Puffed wheat, puffed rice, and cornflakes may be light on calories, but as low-fiber, high-glycemic foods, they send blood sugar through the roof, says Dr. Lieberman. Choose an unsweetened cereal that contains at least 3 grams of fiber per serving, such as Nabisco Shredded Wheat.

Pick beans. Dried beans score low on the glycemic index and are an excellent source of protein, says Dr. Lieberman. While virtually all dried beans are also a good source of fiber, black-eyed peas, chickpeas, kidney beans, lima beans, and black beans are fiber champs, containing 6 to 8 grams of fiber in a ½-cup serving.

Yam it up. Sweet potatoes have a lower glycemic index than white potatoes, so enjoy them often, says Dr. Lieberman. They're great mashed, for example. Or, for mouthwatering "fries," slice sweet potatoes into thin strips, coat them with a tablespoon of olive oil and a sprinkling of paprika, and bake them at 400°F for 40 minutes.

Make mixed-up meals. Consume high-glycemic foods, such as white rice, with a high-protein food, such as chicken. The mix of carbohydrates and protein will keep your blood sugar from rising too quickly, which will slow your body's release of insulin.

The Fat Factor

Is there any woman who doesn't slow down when she wheels her shopping cart past a display of sticky buns?

If you need a good reason to keep walking, here it is: Eating less pastry and other foods high in saturated fat can help us maintain or increase our levels of youth hormones, according to Dr. Giampapa.

On the other hand, a steady diet of saturated fat switches off production of hGH, IGF-1, and DHEA. "We don't know why saturated fat has this effect, but it does," says Dr. Kogan.

We can encourage our bodies' production of youth hormones by getting no more than 10 percent of our daily calories from saturated fat, says Dr. Giampapa. In other words, if you consume 1,800 calories a day, no more than 180 of them (about 16 to 20 grams) should come from saturated fat.

As you trim the saturated fats from your diet, replace them with foods high in monounsaturated fats, such as nuts, avocados, and canola, olive, and peanut oils, says Dr. Giampapa.

Monounsaturated fats tend to reduce low-density lipoprotein (LDL) cholesterol and raise high-density lipoprotein (HDL) cholesterol. That's not only good for our hearts, it's good for our youth hormone levels, too. The higher our HDL levels, the better equipped our bodies are to make DHEA, estrogen, and testosterone, says Dr. Giampapa. (That's because these particular hormones are actually made from cholesterol.)

Olive oil is perhaps the best-known monounsaturated fat. And it can do more than lower LDL cholesterol. It contains several compounds, such as polyphenols, that are powerful antioxidants. These substances keep the LDL cholesterol in our bloodstream from being damaged by free radicals, making it less likely to stick to artery walls.

The Zorba Diet

Fish, nuts, olive oil . . . Zorba the Greek would have no problem getting 30 percent of his daily calories from monounsaturated fats, as Dr. Giampapa suggests. The tips below can help you eat like Zorba.

Go a little nutty. The people in Mediterranean countries eat a lot of nuts, a primo source of monounsaturated fats. Follow their example and toss a small handful of raw almonds, walnuts, or sunflower or pumpkin seeds on salads, rice dishes, or veggies, suggests Dr. Lieberman. In a 10-year study of 86,016 women ages 34 to 59 conducted by researchers at the Harvard School of Public Health, women who ate 5 ounces of nuts a week were 35 percent less likely to have heart disease, most likely because of the nuts' beneficial effects on cholesterol.

Get hooked on fish. Eat fish such as salmon, tuna, cod, haddock, herring, perch, or

WOMEN ASK WHY

If bean curd is so good for you, why does it sound so bad?

There's no denying it. Bean curd, more commonly called tofu, has a bad rep in this country. Perhaps the phrase *bean curd* conjures up a vision of curdled milk. But despite the negative impressions that this soy-derived food inspires, its health benefits are quite positive.

Research shows, for example, that soy is rich in antioxidants, specifically genistein and daidzin. Antioxidants help reduce the negative effects of free radicals—unstable oxygen molecules that damage cells and contribute to many age-related health problems in this country, such as heart disease and cancer. It's noteworthy that people in Japan and China, who tend to consume diets high in soy, are less likely to develop these serious diseases. And American women may be interested to know that Asian women going through menopause seem to experience fewer hot flashes.

Tofu is an excellent source of high-quality protein, and it is a good source of other beneficial nutrients, such as iron, calcium, and potassium. But unlike the protein in meat and dairy products, it contains no cholesterol and only a small amount of saturated fat.

People may believe that tofu has an unpleasant taste, but actually, tofu has virtually no taste at all. This blandness actually works in its favor, because it takes on the flavor of anything it's cooked with. For example, you can hide soft tofu in soups, sauces, and desserts. And firm tofu can be grilled, added to soups and stews, or fried in olive or canola oil.

Expert consulted
John H. Weisburger, Ph.D., M.D.
Senior member
American Health Foundation
Valhalla, New York

snapper once or twice a week, suggests Dr. Lieberman. These fish, caught in the deepest and coldest waters of the North Atlantic, are rich in omega-3 fatty acids, substances that

THE BULB OF LONG LIFE

Suddenly realizing that your breath smells of garlic ranks near the top of our Most Mortifying Moments index. But from a scientific standpoint, reeking of garlic is a *good* thing.

Why? Research suggests that the powerful chemicals that make our breath reek may also help us live longer.

"Garlic has so many anti-aging properties," says Alexander G. Schauss, Ph.D., director of natural and medical products research at the American Institute for Biosocial Research in Tacoma, Washington. "That's because it prevents or treats many illnesses that shorten life span, such as cardiovascular disease and cancer."

Garlic has been found to thin the blood and lower cholesterol, which can help prevent the blood vessel problems that can lead to high blood pressure, heart disease, and stroke, says Dr. Schauss.

While recent research has cast doubt on garlic's cholesterol-fighting abilities, critics say that the garlic powder and garlic oil used in those studies may not have contained the bulb's cholesterol-lowering compounds.

Garlic also seems to help prevent cancer. Population studies have found that people in garlic-loving countries such as Italy and China tend to develop less gastrointestinal cancers—those that affect the mouth, esophagus, stomach, colon, and rectum, says Dr. Schauss.

Consuming just two to four cloves a day can help prevent and treat disease, according to research conducted by Dr. Schauss.

Garlic is so versatile that you can throw a few cloves into virtually any dish, from spaghetti sauce, soups, and stews to stir-fried vegetables. Or roast it, which gives garlic a sweet, caramelized flavor. Simply cut the top from the garlic bulb to expose the tips of the cloves, rub with a little olive oil, wrap in foil, and bake for 45 minutes at 350°F.

Important: After you chop or crush garlic, let it stand for 15 to 20 minutes, says Dr. Schauss. According to recent studies, immediately cooking garlic after it has been chopped or crushed can reduce or eliminate its healing properties. Letting garlic sit allows enough time for oxygen to react with the chemicals in garlic to form the therapeutic substance allicin.

have been shown to raise HDL cholesterol. (Omega-3's also help make eicosanoids, hormonelike substances that encourage our bodies to make hGH, says Dr. Giampapa.)

Feast on a fatty fruit. Toss a few chunks of avocado into your salads, or add a few slices to a sandwich in place of cheese. Avocados are rich in oleic acid, the same monounsaturated fat found in olive oil. Since avocados are high in calories and contain about 30 grams of fat apiece, enjoy them in moderation, says Dr. Lieberman.

Protect olive oil. Buy small bottles of olive oil with long, narrow necks. And after you use the oil, cap the bottle tightly and refrigerate it. "These steps limit the oil's exposure to oxygen, which will keep it from turning rancid and discourage the formation of free radicals," says Robert Goldman, D.O., Ph.D., cofounder of the American Academy of Anti-Aging Medicine and coauthor of *Stopping the Clock*.

Refrigerated olive oil will solidify. When you're ready to use it, run the bottle under warm water for a few minutes, then pour off the reliquefied oil that forms at the top.

What about Meat?

Just like Mom always said, meat is an excellent source of protein. And what was good for you when you were growing up is still good for you now that you're growing older.

Our bodies use the protein in

meat and other high-protein foods to make amino acids. These substances help our bodies make their own proteins, which are used to regulate hormones, grow new tissue, and repair or replace worn-out tissue.

Unfortunately, meat tends to be high in saturated fat. So you may be wondering: If I cut back on meat, will I lose out on protein? No, says Dr. Giampapa. We can get the protein we need from food without consuming meat at all.

A wide array of plant foods, including beans and grains, are excellent sources of protein, says Dr. Lieberman. Some, such as soy and the grain quinoa (pronounced "KEEN-wah"), are considered "complete" proteins because they contain all of the nine essential amino acids we need to stay healthy. But our bodies will make their own complete proteins if we eat enough calories and a variety of plant foods, such as nuts and seeds, grains, and fruits and vegetables.

Get the Protein, Forgo the Fat

The bottom line? It's absolutely okay to eat meat as long as you don't eat Fred Flintstone–size portions every day and you get the majority of your protein from plant sources, says Dr. Lieberman. Here's how to get the protein you need without the saturated fat.

Toss back a soy cocktail. Soy foods such as soy milk and tofu are an excellent source of protein. But if you don't enjoy these foods, drink one of the great-tasting soy shakes available in health food stores, suggests Dr. Lieberman. "They're a great way to consume high-quality protein every day or a few times a week."

Before you select a soy shake, read its label, advises Gregory Burke, M.D., professor and interim chairperson in the department of public health sciences at Wake Forest University School of Medicine in Winston-Salem, North Carolina. While some brands are low in fat and contain natural sweeteners, others are loaded with sugar and fat.

Get keen on quinoa. The beadlike, ivory-colored seeds of this plant are usually eaten like rice. But you can also cook it in fruit juice and eat it for breakfast, use it as a substitute for rice in pudding, or make a cold salad of quinoa, beans, and chopped vegetables. Its soft texture and somewhat bland flavor make it easy to add to other foods, such as soups and pasta dishes. You'll find quinoa in health food stores.

Use the palm computer. To avoid eating too much meat at any one meal, use this simple guideline of Dr. Giampapa's: Don't eat more meat than you can fit in the palm of your hand. And aim to eat four handfuls of vegetables to every one handful of fish or lean meat.

Wok meat into your diet. Adding a small amount of steak or pork to a vegetable stir-fry lets you savor the flavor of meat for a fraction of its saturated fat and calories, says Dr. Lieberman.

The Toxic Avengers

Free radicals hit our bodies 10,000 times a day. Adding injury to injury, these little molecules actually burn holes through the membranes that surround cells, the better to penetrate and vanquish them.

Faced with this onslaught of malicious marauders, hell-bent on crippling our cells and mutating our cellular DNA, our bodies could use a little help. That's where antioxidants come in. These common vitamins such as C and E and minerals such as zinc and selenium neutralize free radicals.

So do phytochemicals, substances in common fruits, vegetables, and other plant foods. Phytochemicals also seem to fight a plethora of age-related diseases, from arthritis to cancer.

To give just a few examples, ellagic acid, a compound found in berries (with strawberries and blackberries containing the most), may help prevent cellular changes that can lead to cancer. Lutein, found in dark green vegetables like spinach and kale, has been found to cut the risk of macular degeneration nearly in half. Indole-3 carbinol, found in broccoli, cabbage, and other cruciferous vegetables, may help prevent breast and cervical cancer.

In short, every juicy berry, steamed broccoli floret, or spinach salad we consume helps sheath our bodies in nutritional armor to stem free-radical damage and help prevent age-related disease.

Great Ways to Ambush Radicals

The way we choose, store, and cook antioxidant-rich fruits and vegetables can boost their protective effect. Here's how to get the most from their anti-aging powers.

Choose the antioxidant allstars. Wondering which vegetables will give you the most antioxidant bang for your buck? Wonder no more. Researchers at the Jean Mayer USDA Human Nutrition Research Center on Aging at Tufts University in Boston analyzed 22 common vegetables, then calculated the ability of each to neutralize free radicals. The winners included kale, beets, red bell peppers, brussels sprouts, broccoli florets, potatoes, sweet potatoes, and corn.

Follow Popeye's lead. Consider eating more spinach and strawberries, too. Their high levels of antioxidants may prevent or even re-

WOMAN TO WOMAN
Going Vegetarian Sparked Her Youth

For 13 years, Mary Jane Soares tried every conceivable type of diet to control the health conditions that were sapping her youthful energy. Now at 48, this registered nurse in Emeryville, California, has found a way of eating that has improved her health and helped her regain her zest for life.

In 1982, I began getting sick when I ate certain foods, especially if they contained sugar or wheat. And I was exhausted all the time. It was a chore just to get up in the morning. I was 31 and feeling ancient.

I went to a doctor, who diagnosed me with a triple whammy—food allergies, yeast infection, and chronic fatigue syndrome. I was put on various elimination diets—no wheat or sugar, just fruits and vegetables, meat, and a few grains—to discover which foods I couldn't eat.

I ate this way and felt good until 1984, when I moved from Little Rock, Arkansas, to California. I thought I could continue the diet on my own. But I splurged too much on sugar and started getting sick again. Truthfully, I never really got well.

For the next 10 years, I tried a variety of treatments to control my health problems, from homeopathy to supplementation programs. Nothing helped much.

In 1997, I found a new doctor, who did some tests and found undigested protein in my blood, which meant that I was not digesting my food properly. He prescribed medication and supplements. In search of a more natural remedy, I then went to a nutritionist. She started me on an intensive detoxification program and encouraged me to become a vegetarian.

So I did.

verse the effects of free-radical damage to the brain, helping to keep it sharp as we age, according to another study conducted at the USDA Human Nutrition Research Center on Aging at Tufts University.

Since then, I've never felt better. I have fruit in the morning and a midmorning snack of organic raw almond butter on some flaxseed crackers. Lunch is usually vegetables—my favorites are broccoli, pea pods, and asparagus, when it's in season. Or I'll have potato-and-leek soup. Dinner is more vegetables and, occasionally, salmon.

As good as I feel, it's hard to not be able to eat everything I want, especially to a sugarholic like me. What saved me is my love for cooking. I wasn't going to eat steamed vegetables, baked potatoes, and salad all my life without at least trying to make them interesting and tasty. I learned to make things such as vegetarian sushi rolls, creamed curried squash soup made with almond milk, and sherbets made from fresh frozen fruit. To calm my sweet tooth, I mash up butternut squash and sprinkle it with cinnamon and an herbal sweetener called stevia.

Since I eat virtually no meat, I get the majority of my protein through nuts and seeds. I love almonds—sometimes I eat them like M&Ms, a handful at a time. Or I grind them and make a pâté that I put in my vegetarian sushi rolls. I get my calcium primarily through green vegetables and in my multivitamin/mineral supplement. I just had a bone-density scan this last year, and my bones are strong and healthy.

I feel strong and healthy, too. My candida is under control—so much so that once a month or so, I can splurge and have a piece of chocolate cake without feeling ill.

And I've got energy to burn. When I started this way of eating, I was able to jump on my mini-trampoline for 2 minutes. Now I can do it for 20 to 30 minutes at a clip. I've even started snowboarding. I just feel more alive and vibrant. And, yes, younger.

This way of eating allows me to live life the way it should be lived—to the fullest.

Researchers fed 344 test animals extracts of strawberry or spinach, vitamin E, or a control diet. After 8 months, they tested the rats' long- and short-term memories. The rats that consumed the daily equivalent of a large spinach salad performed better when made to run a maze than those fed a normal diet, strawberry extract, or vitamin E. However, the spinach and strawberry extracts and the vitamin E diet all slowed signs of aging in the rats in other tests. The spinach extract, in particular, is speculated to have protected different types of nerve cells in various parts of the brain against the effects of aging.

Choose high-octane olive oil. Cold-pressed, extra-virgin olive oil contains more antioxidants and phytochemicals than yellow olive oil, says Dr. Lieberman. That's because it is extracted by literally crushing the olives, rather than by using heat and chemicals.

Don't be put off by this oil's greenish hue. "Yellow olive oil is yellow because it's been processed and heated, which removes all the good stuff," says Dr. Lieberman. While you'll pay more for extra-virgin oil, it's healthier (and, according to many folks, tastier) than less expensive varieties.

Seek the color purple. If you see broccoli that's so dark it's almost purple, put it in your shopping cart. That purply color means it's packing a mother lode of beta-carotene. If it's yellow, don't buy it—it's lost its vital nutrients.

Quick-cook veggies. Steam rather than boil your vegetables, advises Dr. Lieberman. "Steaming locks in their antioxidants and phytonutrients," she says. When you boil them, you leave their protective substances in the water.

Simplify salad prep. No time to peel, slice, and dice salad fixings? Do it once a week, suggests Dr. Giampapa. Every Sunday, prepare a huge bowl of dark green lettuce, along with carrots, peppers, and other fixings. Store them separately in airtight plastic bags or containers to limit their exposure to oxygen.

Is That a Toxin in My "Soup"?

As we mentioned earlier, our cells are filled with a broth of nutrients and other substances called cytoplasm. It's where the action is—where cellular machinery makes energy, synthesizes proteins, and disarms free radicals.

It's hard for cells to get the fuel they need to perform these important jobs from the typical American diet, say anti-aging experts. Foods high in fat and sugar and processed foods containing additives and preservatives sic free radicals on our hapless bodies. These chemicals build up in our bodies, gradually weakening our cellular machinery.

What's more, sugary, fatty foods laced with preservatives and additives tend to turn to acid in our blood, upsetting our bodies' delicate pH balance, says Dr. Giampapa. A steady diet of them acidifies our cellular soup, causing cells and tissues to age before their time.

Just as cars run smoother and cleaner on high-octane fuel, we run best on foods that don't contain additives and preservatives and that keep our bodies close to a neutral pH, says Dr. Giampapa. These foods are—you guessed it—fruits, vegetables, legumes, and whole grains.

Put Your Diet into Rehab

The cleaner and more natural our diets, the more nutrients our cells get—and the more efficiently they are likely to work, says Dr. Giampapa. The strategies below can help put your diet into detox.

Eat naked produce. Make an effort to buy organic fruits and vegetables (those grown without these chemicals) whenever you can, says Dr. Goldman. It's easier to find organic produce than it used to be, he says. "Many supermarkets now carry organic fruits and vegetables alongside the commercially grown variety, and some food chains (such as Fresh Fields, Bread and Circus, and Whole Food Markets) carry only organic food." Make sure that you wash organic produce to remove as much bacteria and dirt as possible.

Buy boxed organics. If you can't find organic fruits and vegetables, consider buying other organic products, says Dr. Lieberman. "I buy organic cereal, organic milk, and organic juice and eggs," she says. "If you can get even 20 percent of your diet organic, that's 20 percent less of a toxic burden on your immune system."

Waylay white-sugar cravings. When a craving for a slice of coffee ring or another sugary, fatty food strikes, "eat a cold sweet potato," says Dr. Lieberman. "Its natural sweetness may be enough to satisfy your craving for white sugar." If this trick works for you, bake up a mess of them and have them on hand for those times when you get the "craves."

Soy: Future Youth

Soy is a superfood," says Shari Lieberman, Ph.D., a nutrition scientist and exercise physiologist in New York City. "You might even call it a youth food because it has such potential to stave off age-related conditions from menopausal symptoms to osteoporosis to breast cancer."

Skeptical? Think about the robust health and super-longevity of people in Asian countries, where soy is a dietary staple. Compared to Americans, Asians who eat a traditional soy-rich diet have fewer heart attacks; are less likely to develop breast, colon, and prostate cancers; and suffer fewer hip fractures. Asian women going through menopause don't have as many hot flashes. And the Japanese, as a population, have the longest life expectancies in the world.

Adding soy to your diet is easy. The new generation of soy foods actually tastes good, with none of the beany flavor or unpleasant aftertaste that characterized soy products of the past. Your family will never suspect that you're serving them soy in those delicious new burgers, hot dogs, or sausage or that you're sneaking tofu or soy milk into their favorite dishes. And afterward, you'll feel great for having treated yourself—and your family—to a delectable serving of good health.

Little Bean, Big Benefits

Soy is an excellent source of low-calorie, high-quality protein, a nutrient we need more of as we grow older. Protein builds and repairs tissue and makes infection-fighting antibodies. But unlike the protein in animal foods, such as meat, eggs, and milk, soy protein contains zero heart-damaging saturated fat and cholesterol. Soy is packed with other nutrients that older bodies need, such as iron, calcium, and B vitamins like thiamin, riboflavin, and niacin.

But that's not all. Nestled in the heart of soybeans are substances called isoflavones, which are part of a group of plant substances known as phytochemicals. The isoflavones in soy, called phytoestrogens, may be the key to soy's disease-fighting powers, says Gregory Burke, M.D., professor and interim chairperson in the department of public health sciences at Wake Forest University School of Medicine in Winston-Salem, North Carolina.

WOMAN TO WOMAN
Thanks to Soy, Menopause Is a Breeze

Linda Townsend, 46, was getting hot under the collar about her menopausal symptoms—literally. As a controller for a construction company in Titusville, Florida, she'd often find herself in an important meeting when she'd suddenly experience a debilitating hot flash. Her hot flashes were so noticeable and frequent that people would stop and stare. Her night sweats were so bad that she'd get up two and three times a night to change clothes. Then she found an answer. Here is her story.

I would be sitting there, and out of nowhere I would be flushed.

The hot feeling would start in my chest and work its way up to my neck, then my face. My face would turn red, and I'd sweat like crazy. Not only did the flashes come fast and furious, but they happened all the time. It got to the point where I'd bring an extra shirt to work every day because I'd sweat so bad that the shirt I'd have on would get soaked. The flashes became so noticeable that my boss would sometimes walk in and say, "You're having another one."

For 4 months, I didn't get a good night's sleep. At least twice a night, I'd have to get up and change my nightgown, then try to find a dry spot on the bed.

I didn't get any relief from what my doctor gave me. But I had been reading Dr. Andrew Weil's Web site, and he had recommended soy for hot flashes. I thought about using soy, but for the longest time I couldn't bring myself to do it. To me, even the word *soy* didn't sound good. After reading hundreds of testimonials, though, I finally gave in. I started with a glass of soy milk every day and ate a soy burger every other day or so.

Within 2 weeks, the hot flashes stopped. I couldn't believe it. I thought maybe it wasn't the soy. Maybe they'd stopped on their own. But when I went on a 2-week vacation in Europe where there was no soy available, my flashes came back. The first thing I did when I got home was pour myself a glass of soy milk.

I feel empowered now. I used to think hot flashes were just something I was stuck with, but I was wrong. I've learned how to take control of them.

The average Asian consumes 50 milligrams of isoflavones a day—the amount in 2 to 3 ounces of soy, says Dr. Burke. Consuming these minuscule amounts may afford you the protection that many Asians enjoy from many of the illnesses of aging, including the ones below.

Cancer. In animal and test-tube studies, the phytoestrogen genistein slows the growth of cancer cells. How? Researchers don't know. But they do know that genistein and another phytoestrogen, daidzein, act as weaker versions of the estrogen that women produce naturally.

It is well-known that estrogen can fuel so-called hormone-dependent cancers of the breast and uterus. Dr. Burke says it may be that soy phytoestrogens compete with natural estrogen for molecules on the surfaces of cells that recognize and bind to estrogen. If soy phytoestrogens fill these receptors, the more potent natural estrogen can't, thereby helping to prevent cancer.

High cholesterol. Soy may lower both "bad" low-density lipoprotein (LDL) and total cholesterol levels without reducing "good" high-density lipoprotein (HDL) cholesterol. In one large study conducted at the University of Kentucky, the LDL cholesterol of people who consumed about 2 ounces of soy protein a day plunged 12.9 percent, and their total cholesterol dropped 9.3 percent. Their levels of "good" HDL cholesterol stayed steady.

No one knows exactly how soy might lower cholesterol. But one theory is that soy phytoestrogens help transport LDL cholesterol from the bloodstream to the liver, where it's broken down and excreted. Phytoestrogens may also keep LDL from turning rancid (a process known as oxidation), making it less likely to clog the walls of your arteries.

Osteoporosis. Soy phytoestrogens appear not only to repair bone but actually to build it. In one study, women who consumed 40 grams of soy protein (containing high concentrations of isoflavones) a day for 6 months significantly increased the thickness of the bone in their lower spines. And there's another reason to bone up on soy: Animal protein seems to speed up the body's excretion of calcium. Apparently, soy protein doesn't, says Dr. Burke.

Menopausal symptoms. Sometimes isoflavones block a woman's natural supply of estrogen, and sometimes, they actually supplement it. This is a boon for women in menopause, when declining levels of estrogen and progesterone can trigger hot flashes and night sweats. In one study, women who consumed 60 grams of soy protein a day for 12 weeks cut their rate of hot flashes by nearly half.

Supermarket Soy

By now, the soy revolution has probably reached your supermarket. With tofu in the produce section, soy milk in the dairy case, and soy-based frozen yogurts next to the Häagen-Dazs, it has never been easier to add soy to your diet. But if you haven't yet joined the revolution, read on to get acquainted with these commonly available soy foods.

Tofu. The mother of all soy foods comes in three varieties, one as versatile as the next. Firm tofu is solid, so it's often stir-fried, grilled, or added to soups and stews. Soft tofu, which has a creamy consistency, and silken tofu, which has a custardlike texture, can be mashed or pureed and added to blender drinks, dips, dressings, and puddings. Don't be put off by its taste. Standing alone, tofu is bland, but it takes on the flavors of other foods that it's mixed with.

Tempeh. Pronounced "TEM-pay," this traditional Indonesian food is made of cooked, fermented whole soybeans. The result is a chunky, tender cake with a smoky or nutty flavor. Tempeh is a tasty, low-fat alternative to meat—in fact, many women marinate it and grill it, just like a steak. Tempeh can also be added to soups, casseroles, or chili.

SEARCH OUT SOY "EXOTICS"

When it comes to soy, tofu isn't the only game in town. Explore your local natural foods store or Asian market for the more exotic fare below.

Edamamé. These are large soybeans, harvested when they're still green and sweet. Boil them for 15 to 20 minutes, and you have a high-fiber, high-protein, cholesterol-free, soy-rich snack or main vegetable dish.

Okara. Okara is the pulpy fiber by-product of soy milk. It tastes similar to coconut, so try adding it to baked goods, such as cookies or muffins, or sprinkling it over your breakfast cereal.

Soybeans (whole). As soybeans mature in the pod, they ripen into a hard, dry bean—yellow, black, or brown. Whole soybeans are an excellent source of protein and dietary fiber; add the cooked beans to sauces, stews, and soups.

Soy nuts. This nutty-tasting snack food is actually whole soybeans that have been soaked in water, then roasted. High in protein and a concentrated source of isoflavones, soy nuts are similar in texture and flavor to peanuts. Soy nuts can be found in a variety of flavors, including chocolate-covered.

Soy nut butter. If you're a peanut butter junkie, give this nutty-tasting spread a try. Made from whole, roasted soy nuts, soy nut butter contains significantly less fat than peanut butter.

Soy milk. This creamy liquid comes from soybeans that are soaked, finely ground, and strained. It's a good source of protein and B vitamins, and many brands are fortified with calcium. Lots of folks pour it over their breakfast cereal or use it in cooking. And since soy milk comes in a variety of flavors, including vanilla and chocolate, some folks drink it straight. Because it isn't dairy milk, look for "soy beverage" or "soy drink" on the labels when you are purchasing soy milk.

Sneaking Soy into Your Diet

Many women have come to enjoy soy foods. Others . . . well, it might take a little longer. If you fall into the latter category, take the stealth approach to soy, in which you sneak the stuff into already familiar dishes. These ideas will get you started.

Cook up some pudding. You could get 30 to 50 milligrams of isoflavones by consuming 1 cup of soy milk or ½ cup of tofu or tempeh. Or you could savor some creamy pudding. Pudding mixes are made to be blended with firm tofu. One brand, Mori-Nu, contains 30 milligrams of isoflavones per ½ cup. Or simply add 2 cups of soy milk to your favorite fat-free pudding mix.

Savor a smoothie. For another quick dessert, blend ½ cup silken tofu with ½ cup each fresh berries, nonfat yogurt, and skim milk. Add a dash of vanilla or honey if you like.

Dig into pizza. "Soy can transform pizza from everyone's favorite 'fun' food into serious nutrition," writes Patricia Greenberg in her book *The Whole Soy Cookbook*. Start with a homemade crust that contains soy flour, add tomato sauce and shredded soy mozzarella cheese, then top it with crumbled soy sausage or soy pepperoni. Delicious.

Kick back with a latte. Microwave 1 cup of vanilla soy milk for 60 seconds, then add 1 teaspoon of instant coffee. No need for sugar—vanilla soy milk is sweet. This elegant beverage packs 30 milligrams of isoflavones.

Go nuts. If you're hooked on roasted peanuts, try soy nuts. They are a concentrated source of isoflavones and a tasty, high-protein alternative to other roasted nuts, says Patricia Murphy, Ph.D., professor in the food science and human nutrition department at Iowa State University in Ames. "They taste somewhat like peanuts and make a great snack."

Slip soy into sweets. Bake with soy flour, suggests Dr. Murphy. Just ½ cup contains 30 to 50 milligrams of isoflavones. When baking quick breads and muffins, replace one-quarter to one-third of the total flour with soy flour. In yeast-raised recipes, use only 15 percent soy flour, or just a little more than ⅛ cup. (Soy flour is gluten-free, so expect yeast-raised breads to be denser in texture.)

You can find soy flour in natural food stores. Keep it in the fridge or freezer; soy flour goes bad more quickly than processed white flour.

Play hide-the-tofu. If you're exploring the countless delicious ways to prepare tofu, take a bow. But if you just want to hide the stuff, add cubed tofu to soups, stews, chili, and spaghetti sauce.

Take a powder. Add 2 to 3 tablespoons of powdered isolated soy protein (ISP) to milk, juice, or health shakes, suggests Dr. Burke. Available at health food stores, ISP is a simple way to get soy protein *and* isoflavones. Pass up ready-made soy shakes, however. "They tend to contain a lot of sugar and fat and may not be as healthy as you think," he says.

Get out the ketchup. Try the new breed of soy hot dogs, burgers, and sausage (as well as the many soy cheeses and yogurts), suggests Dr. Burke. While these products contain few or no isoflavones, they are still lower in total and saturated fat and cholesterol than their full-fat counterparts. "And that's still to your benefit," he says.

Time Capsules: The Anti-Aging Supplements

Phosphatidylserine. It doesn't exactly spell P-R-O-M-I-S-I-N-G, does it?

It looks more like one of those unpronounceable ingredients listed on the label of a hair shampoo. But actually, it's brimming with promise. This natural supplement is on the cutting edge of anti-aging medicine. It has been shown to renew brain cells and sharpen mental performance.

Where can you find this exotic stuff? (It's pronounced "foss-fuh-TID-ill-SEER-een," by the way.)

It's sitting on a shelf at your local health food store or just a click away on the Internet, along with other exciting, cutting-edge anti-aging substances that you may not know much about yet. Among them are alpha-lipoic acid, coenzyme Q_{10}, and melatonin, to name just a few.

"I'm sure these supplements seem somewhat mysterious," says Ronald Klatz, M.D., D.O., author of *Brain Fitness* and president of the American Academy of Anti-Aging Medicine, a Chicago-based society of physicians and scientists who believe aging is not inevitable. "After all, we've known about the role of vi-

tamin C in good health for the past 30 years, and vitamin E for longer than that. These are quite new."

What makes these substances so special?

For one thing, many of them are potent antioxidants, says Dr. Klatz. Only antioxidants can neutralize free radicals, the unstable oxygen molecules that punch holes in cell membranes, destroy vital enzymes, damage cellular DNA—and, ultimately, lead to the diseases of aging.

For another, their antioxidant power is, in some cases, many times more powerful than better-known antioxidants such as vitamins C and E. Some actually recycle vitamins C and E, giving them new life in the endless war against free radicals. Still others dissolve in both fat and water, enabling them to neutralize free radicals wherever they occur, from our watery blood to our fatty brains.

These new substances have the potential to extend life span and stave off age-related degenerative diseases, says Dr. Klatz. Future youth is out there!

To decide whether these supplements might be of any benefit to you, here's a primer on some that have longevity experts and medical researchers buzzing.

Alpha-Lipoic Acid (ALA)

What it is: An antioxidant made by the body, ALA also helps break down food into the energy needed by your cells. It helps the body recycle and renew vitamins C and E, making them serviceable again. And unlike many antioxidants, which dissolve only in fat or only in water, ALA fights free radicals in both the fatty and watery parts of cells, protecting both from free-radical damage. "Lipoic acid can zip in and out of any cell in the body, even those in the brain," says Lester Packer, Ph.D., professor of molecular and cell biology at the University of California, Berkeley.

How it delays aging: Clinical studies suggest that ALA may help prevent the nerve damage, caused by free-radical attacks, that frequently accompanies diabetes. In one German study, intravenous ALA significantly reduced pain, tingling, and numbness in the feet of people with diabetes.

What you'll find: ALA comes in capsules and tablets, in dosages from 50 to 300 milligrams.

How much to take: The general recommended dose is 50 to 100 milligrams a day. In the treatment of diabetes, the recommended dosage is 300 to 600 milligrams a day, says Dr. Packer.

Be aware: If you have diabetes and are being treated for symptoms of nerve damage, Dr. Packer suggests that you talk to your doctor before taking ALA supplements.

DON'T FORGET YOUR MULTI

"A multivitamin/mineral supplement is the cornerstone of any smart supplement regimen," says Jeffrey Blumberg, Ph.D., chief of the antioxidants research laboratory at the U.S.D.A. Human Nutrition Research Center on Aging at Tufts University in Boston.

But how can you know if the multi you are taking is a good one? Read the label. Look for a multi supplement that contains 100 percent of the Daily Value (DV) for most essential vitamins and minerals. None contains them all. The label should also have the letters USP on it. This stands for United States Pharmacopeia. Also, check the expiration date and don't buy more than you can use before then.

Your multi should contain these essential nutrients.

VITAMINS

Nutrient: Vitamin A or preformed Vitamin A (beta-carotene)

Daily Value: 5,000 international units (IU)

What it does: Helps your eyes adjust to dim light; maintains immunity; and forms and maintains normal structure and function of the epithelial cells (cells that act as a barrier between your body and the environment) in your mouth, eyes, skin, hair, gums, and various glands

Nutrient: Vitamin B_6

Daily Value: 2 milligrams

What it does: Helps your body make red blood cells; helps maintain your immune system; and helps produce insulin (the hormone that aids in converting food to energy)

Nutrient: Vitamin D

Daily Value: 400 IU

What it does: Helps bones mineralize properly by transporting bone-building calcium and phosphorus to the blood and, eventually, to the bones

Nutrient: Folic acid (folate)

Daily Value: 400 micrograms

What it does: Helps you produce DNA and RNA, the genetic code for cell reproduction. It is needed to form hemoglobin, which carries oxygen in red blood cells.

MINERALS

Nutrient: Chromium

Daily Value: 120 micrograms

What it does: Helps your body convert carbohydrates and fats into energy; works with insulin to help your body use glucose (blood sugar)

Nutrient: Copper

Daily Value: 2 milligrams

What it does: Helps your body make hemoglobin, which carries oxygen in red blood cells; and helps your body absorb iron

Nutrient: Iron

Daily Value: 18 milligrams

What it does: Carries oxygen in your blood and removes carbon dioxide, which is formed as your body produces energy; helps protect against infection. Multis come in regular or low- or no-iron formulas. If you have heavy periods, aim for the DV; otherwise, you should look for a multi that contains low or no iron.

Nutrient: Magnesium

Daily Value: 400 milligrams (The most you'll find in a regular multi is 100 milligrams; adding more would make the multi too big to swallow.)

What it does: Helps your body make proteins; helps maintain the cells in your nerves and muscles; plays a role in the mineralization of bones and immune-system function

Nutrient: Selenium

Daily Value: 70 micrograms (Most multis contain less; look for a minimum of 10 micrograms.)

What it does: Works with vitamin E to protect cells from damage by free radicals, unstable oxygen molecules thought to speed up the aging process by damaging our cells and tissues

Nutrient: Zinc

Daily Value: 15 milligrams

What it does: Helps keep your immune system strong; promotes cell reproduction; and helps heal wounds. It is crucial for sperm production and fetal development.

Bioflavonoids

What it is: Bioflavonoids are a group of plant pigments that give fruits and flowers some of their color. Some bioflavonoids act as powerful antioxidants, "many of which are more potent than better-known antioxidants such as vitamins C and E," explains Shari Lieberman, Ph.D., a nutrition scientist and exercise physiologist in New York City.

How it delays aging: Bioflavonoids may help lower the risk of heart disease. In 1996, a Finnish study found that women who ate the most flavonoids had a 46 percent lower risk for heart disease than those who ate the least.

Bioflavonoids keep the tiny disks in our blood (called platelets), which help blood clot, from clumping together and forming clots that can block the arteries. They also keep harmful low-density lipoprotein (LDL) cholesterol from oxidizing and sticking to artery walls.

Some bioflavonoids can stop cancer before it starts. To give just a few examples, quercetin, found in apples, yellow and red onions, and tea, has been shown in test-tube studies to discourage the growth of tumors and prevent malignant cells from spreading. And rutin, found in buckwheat, helps reduce cancer risk through its action as an antioxidant.

What you'll find: You can get bioflavonoids by eating fruits and vegetables or by taking them in supplement form. Supplements may contain either a single bioflavonoid or several in combination, says Michael Janson, M.D., president of the American College for Advancement in Medicine and author of three books including *Dr. Janson's Vitamin Revolution*. These usually contain extracts of quercetin, hesperidin, rutin, and citrus bioflavonoids and come in 500- or 1,000-milligram doses.

How much to take: Dr. Janson recommends taking 1,000 milligrams once or twice a day. As powerful antioxidants themselves, bioflavonoids increase the absorption of vitamin C.

Be aware: They are generally regarded as safe.

Coenzyme Q$_{10}$

What it is: An antioxidant made by our bodies, coenzyme Q$_{10}$ helps make ATP (adenosine triphosphate), the fuel that allows our cells to do their jobs. Every cell in our bodies contains this antioxidant, but it's most concentrated in heart muscle cells, which require the most fuel. We have plenty of coenzyme Q$_{10}$ until we hit age 40. After that, our levels take a nosedive.

How it delays aging: Coenzyme Q$_{10}$ may help prevent or treat many common forms of heart disease, says Peter Langsjoen, M.D., a staff cardiologist at Mother Francis Hospital and the East Texas Medical Center in Tyler. "It provides such dramatic improvement, it's unthinkable for me to practice medicine without it."

Research shows that people with various types of heart disease are deficient in coenzyme Q$_{10}$, and that the more severe the heart disease, the lower these levels drop. This substance appears

to improve the heart's ability to contract. And because it's a powerful antioxidant, coenzyme Q$_{10}$ also helps prevent "bad" LDL cholesterol from sticking to the walls of the arteries and clogging blood vessels.

Coenzyme Q$_{10}$ is used to treat a variety of

clothing and a broad-brimmed hat, slather herself with a sunscreen, spend as much time as possible under an umbrella, and get out of the sun completely for 15 to 20 minutes every hour.

Whatever sunscreen Terri uses should be applied ½ hour before exposure. She could opt for a product that contains a physical sunblock, such as zinc oxide or titanium dioxide. These substances prevent two types of the sun's ultraviolet (UV) rays—UVA and UVB—from being absorbed by the skin.

Or Terri could use what's called a broad-spectrum sunscreen. An active ingredient in these products, avobenzone, also known as Parsol 1789, blocks both UVA and UVB rays.

Whatever product Terri uses, it should have a sun protection factor (SPF) of at least 15. Because her skin is so fair, she should reapply it every few hours, whether she thinks she needs it or not. And she needs to remember that as protective as sunscreen is, it still allows some UV rays to penetrate skin. During her "sun breaks," Terri should also check to see if her skin is turning pink, a sign that she's on her way to a skin-damaging sunburn. If her skin is turning pink, she should get out of the sun for the rest of the day.

As for becoming a "bronzed beachcomber," the brown of a real tan means that the skin has already been damaged and at some point may shown signs of premature aging and skin cancer. If sun-kissed is the look Terri really wants, the artificial tanning oil will give it to her without any sun exposure at all.

Expert consulted
Karen Keller, M.D.
Dermatologist
Burlingame, California

opathy conducted by Dr. Langsjoen, those who took 100 milligrams of coenzyme Q_{10} a day along with their conventional therapy did far better than those who got conventional therapy and a placebo.

Coenzyme Q_{10} also helps treat congestive heart failure, which occurs when the heart is too weak to pump blood through the body. In a large study conducted by Dr. Langsjoen, 58 percent of people taking coenzyme Q_{10} improved by one New York Heart Association classification (the standard doctors use to assess heart patients' condition), 28 percent improved by two classes, and 43 percent stopped using one or more drugs.

What you'll find: Coenzyme Q_{10} can be found in 10- to 200-milligram capsules. Dr. Langsjoen prefers the soft-gel supplements prepared with oil because they're better absorbed by the body.

How much to take: As a preventive measure, take from 30 to 60 milligrams per day, says Dr. Langsjoen. He prescribes higher doses—120 to 360 milligrams—for people with heart problems.

This nutrient dissolves only in the presence of fat, so if you're using coenzyme Q_{10} supplements that aren't in gel form, take them with a meal or snack that contains a small amount of fat, says Dr. Langsjoen.

Be aware: Some medications deplete the body's supply of coenzyme Q_{10}. These include cholesterol-lowering drugs such as lovastatin (Mevacor). In rare occurrences, a slight decrease in the effectiveness of the blood thinner warfarin (Coumadin) has been observed. Also, if you

heart conditions, from heart pain (angina) to cardiomyopathy (any noninflammatory disease of the heart muscles). Some studies suggest that this antioxidant helps treat angina by allowing heart muscle cells to use oxygen more efficiently. In a small study of 19 people with cardiomyhave heart disease, consult your doctor before taking coenzyme Q$_{10}$, says Dr. Langsjoen.

Flaxseed Oil

What it is: A polyunsaturated vegetable oil that's a rich source of omega-3 fatty acids. Studies have repeatedly suggested that omega-3's lower blood levels of cholesterol and triglycerides and reduce the stickiness of platelets, thus reducing the risk of heart attack or stroke. Other studies have found that omega-3's raise high-density lipoproteins (HDLs), the "good" cholesterol that helps whisk artery-clogging LDL out of the blood. While fish oils are the best-known sources of omega-3's, flaxseed oil contains twice the amount of omega-3's as fish oils do.

How it delays aging: Researchers have conducted numerous studies on flaxseed to study its potential in preventing and treating cancer, particularly breast and colon cancer. In animal studies, flaxseed helps keep breast cancer from starting and slows the growth of breast tumors already in place.

Research suggests that the cancer-fighting substance in flaxseed is lignan precursors, compounds that the body converts into lignans. These are estrogen-like compounds that may prevent breast cancer by taking up estrogen receptors on breast cells, thereby blocking stronger, cancer-causing estrogen.

Lignans also act as antioxidants and contain other beneficial plant chemicals. An accumulating body of research suggests that they may help protect against age-related chronic conditions such as heart disease.

What you'll find: There are a wide variety of flaxseed oils on the market, but not all are equally beneficial, notes Michael T. Murray, N.D., a faculty member at Bastyr University in Kenmore, Washington, in his book *Understanding Fats and Oils.*

He recommends choosing a brand that has been processed using a technique called modified atmospheric packing (MAP). This method squeezes the oil from the seed at low temperatures while also protecting it from the damaging effects of light and oxygen. Some trade names for MAP processing include Bio-Electron Process, used by Barlean's Organic Oils; SpectraVac Cold-Pressed, used by Spectrum Naturals; and the Omegaflo process, used by Omega Nutrition.

Because lignan precursors are found only in the hull of flaxseeds, many brands of flaxseed oil don't contain these beneficial compounds. Some brands that do are Barlean's Organic High-Lignan Flaxseed Oil, Spectrum Naturals' High-Lig Flax Oil, and Hi-Lignan Flax Seed Oil from Omega Nutrition. They are available in some health food stores or by mail order.

One more thing: Buy only those brands that come in light-resistant plastic containers. Light causes any oil, including flaxseed oil, to break down and turn rancid.

How much to take: Take 1 tablespoon per 100 pounds of body weight a day, suggests Dr. Murray.

Keep flaxseed oil in the freezer until you open it. This will keep its beneficial substances intact. After you open it, keep it in the refrigerator. Also, take flaxseed oil with food (perhaps mix it into yogurt). Your body will absorb and use its essential fatty acids more efficiently. Flaxseed is easily damaged by heat, so don't use it in cooking.

Be aware: Due to its high calorie content, you could gain weight if you don't figure flaxseed oil into your total calorie intake.

Ginkgo

What it is: Ginkgo is an herb extracted from the fan-shaped, leathery leaves of the ginkgo tree.

How it delays aging: This herb helps the brain function more efficiently. Already used in Germany to treat dementia, ginkgo enhances blood circulation, so more nutrients reach brain cells, enabling them to work more efficiently. In European studies, ginkgo has also been found to improve mental performance and short-term memory.

While there's no proof that taking ginkgo now will prevent Alzheimer's disease later, a growing body of research suggests that a concentrated extract of this herb improves the mental functioning of people who already have the disease.

In one of the biggest studies, researchers found that among people with Alzheimer-type dementia and those with dementia caused by blood vessel disease of the brain, those taking ginkgo were better able to think and interact with others than were those taking a placebo.

What you'll find: Ginkgo usually comes in 40-, 60-, or 120-milligram capsules.

How much to take: Take from 120 to 240 milligrams a day in two or three separate doses, says Varro E. Tyler, Ph.D., Sc.D., dean emeritus of the Purdue University School of Pharmacy and Pharmacal Sciences and author of *The Honest Herbal.* The supplement you buy should contain 24 percent flavone glycosides and 6 percent terpenes, says Dr. Tyler. (You might see "24⁄6" on the label.)

Be aware: According to Dr. Tyler, you should be cautious about using ginkgo if you are taking

ARE HORMONE SUPPLEMENTS SAFE?

Some of the anti-aging hormones normally made by your body are now available in bottles at your local health food store. And while the government classifies these "bottled hormones" as dietary supplements, some experts say that they shouldn't be.

"These products are powerful substances and should be viewed as drugs," says Alan R. Gaby, M.D., professor of nutrition at Bastyr University in Kenmore, Washington. "They have potential for great benefit, but they can also cause significant harm."

One example is DHEA (dehydroepiandrosterone). In animal studies, this male hormone (which a woman's body makes, too) appears to boost immunity and help protect against diabetes, heart disease, and even cancer.

Here's the problem. Our bodies convert DHEA into estrogen and testosterone. So if even a small amount is converted to estrogen in a woman with a family history of breast cancer, she may be increasing her risk of developing the disease, says Dr. Gaby.

Pregnenolone, the precursor to DHEA, is another bottled hormone that's flying off the shelves. But clinical research on this hormone is sparse. "There's an animal study that suggests that it improves memory, and that's about it," says Dr. Gaby.

In the body, pregnenolone may be converted into DHEA, increasing our bodies' amounts of estrogen and testosterone. There are potential risks in using pregnenolone, says Dr. Gaby. It hasn't been used long enough to determine if it is safe.

The bottom line: Don't self-prescribe hormone supplements, says Dr. Gaby. Consult a doctor, who will advise you if hormone supplements are appropriate, prescribe them at the appropriate dosage (if necessary), and monitor your progress.

herbs that help prevent blood clotting such as garlic, ginger, and feverfew. Also, don't take it if you're currently using aspirin, warfarin (Coumadin), or an MAO inhibitor drug.

Melatonin

What it is: Melatonin is a hormone secreted by a pea-size gland, called the pineal gland. The hormone helps regulate our sleep patterns. Our levels of melatonin peak by the time we are 3 years old and remain at high levels until after middle age.

How it delays aging: Melatonin is a powerful antioxidant, says Russel J. Reiter, Ph.D., a cellular biologist at the University of Texas Health Science Center at San Antonio, author of *Your Body's Natural Wonder Drug: Melatonin*, and editor of the *Journal of Pineal Research*.

"Melatonin is one of the most powerful antioxidants there is," says Dr. Reiter. As such, it protects against age-related diseases such as cardiovascular disease and cancer, which may be linked to free-radical damage.

But there's more. Unlike many other antioxidants, melatonin is able to cross what's called the blood-brain barrier, which means that it penetrates the brain more easily than some other antioxidants, says Dr. Reiter. So it's better able to fight the free-radical damage in the brain.

Recent evidence suggests that melatonin may also slow the progression of Alzheimer's disease. "Much of the dementia associated with aging, including Alzheimer's disease, is due to loss of neurons as a result of free-radical damage," says Dr. Reiter. "While very high doses of vitamin E, a well-known antioxidant, given for long periods of time can slightly delay Alzheimer's, a recent study on a pair of identical twins found that as little as 6 milligrams of melatonin taken every day for 3 years substantially reduced the progression of Alzheimer's disease."

In some laboratory studies, melatonin has also been found to prevent the growth of cancer cells and to slow the growth of some tumors.

What you'll find: Melatonin usually comes in 3-milligram capsules and tablets. While less common, you can find them in 1-milligram and 0.5-milligram (or 500-microgram) doses as well. Avoid so-called natural melatonin supplements, which probably don't contain enough to be effective, says Dr. Reiter. The synthetic variety, which is probably what you will find, is fine.

How much to take: You take less than you'd think. Although the generally recommended dose is 1 milligram, Dr. Reiter takes 0.5 milligram per day. "And I have the melatonin levels of a young person," he says.

Also, always take melatonin before bed, says Dr. Reiter. And keep your room dark: Darkness stimulates the production of melatonin.

Be aware: Since melatonin makes you drowsy, don't drive or engage in any activity that requires you to be alert after taking it, says Dr. Reiter. Before you start using melatonin, talk with your doctor. Though rare, interactions with prescription medications can occur.

Pycnogenol

What it is: A trademarked supplement derived from the bark of the French maritime pine tree, Pycnogenol (pronounced "pik-NA-je-nal") contains about 40 bioflavonoids with antioxidant powers. Its active ingredients—a class of flavonoids called proanthocyanidins, also found in grape seeds—make it a potent antioxidant. Pycnogenol also recycles vitamin C and, indirectly, vitamin E, making them effective again, says Dr. Packer.

How it delays aging: Pycnogenol reduces the risk of heart disease by keeping platelets unstuck so that they can't adhere to artery walls and by keeping LDL cholesterol from oxidizing, says Dr. Packer.

Pycnogenol also strengthens the body's smallest blood vessels, called capillaries, and prevents free-radical damage to blood vessels. Pycnogenol also suppresses the overproduction of nitric oxide (NO) by immune system cells, which has been linked to rheumatoid arthritis and Alzheimer's disease, says Dr. Packer.

What you'll find: Pycnogenol comes in tablets or capsules, in dosages from 20 milligrams to 100 milligrams.

How much to take: The generally recommended dose is from 50 to 100 milligrams per day, says Dr. Packer.

Phosphatidylserine

What it is: This substance is a phospholipid, a kind of a fat concentrated in the nerve cells of the brain. In elderly people, low levels of phosphatidylserine have been linked with impaired mental functioning and depression.

How it delays aging: Phosphatidylserine improves memory and age-related brain changes, says Timothy Smith, M.D., an expert in anti-aging medicine in Sebastopol, California, and author of *Renewal*. It also helps regenerate damaged nerve cells, so they can send and receive their "messages" more effectively.

Researchers at Stanford University and at Vanderbilt University in Nashville studied the effects of phosphatidylserine in 149 people between the ages of 50 and 75 with "normal" age-related memory loss. The most memory-impaired people reversed an estimated 12-year decline in memory. In other words, the average scores attained by 64-year-olds rose to match the average scores of 52-year-olds.

What you'll find: Phosphatidylserine supplements are made from lecithin, a derivative of soy. In this country, it's available in 20- to 100-milligram capsules and tablets.

How much to take: Dr. Smith recommends taking 100 milligrams of phosphatidylserine two

LIFE EXTENDER
Evade Cancer the One-a-Day Way

Colon cancer is the third most common cancer in women, killing 24,900 of us every year. But taking a daily multivitamin/mineral supplement or a vitamin E supplement may reduce your risk of developing the condition, suggests a study conducted at the Fred Hutchinson Cancer Research Center in Seattle.

Researchers analyzed vitamin use in 444 men and women with colon cancer, focusing on the 10-year period ending 2 years before diagnosis. Then, they compared vitamin use in this group to vitamin use in 426 people without cancer. Researchers found that people who had regularly taken multivitamins for 10 years reduced their risk of colon cancer by 51 percent, and those who took vitamin E may have lowered their risk by 57 percent.

This does not necessarily mean that vitamin supplements are your best protection against cancer. Eating plenty of fruits and vegetables is still the best advice, according to the researchers, because they contain just the right balance of vitamins.

or three times a day. After a month, he says, switch to a maintenance dose of 100 to 200 milligrams a day.

Be aware: Phosphatidylserine appears to be safe with no serious side effects, notes Dr. Smith.

Vitamin C

What it is: An antioxidant nutrient, vitamin C is found in citrus fruits, strawberries, broccoli, kiwifruit, and other fruits and vegetables.

How it delays aging: Studies suggest that people who consume a high-C diet have lower rates of cancer, heart disease, and high blood pressure. There's also evidence that vitamin C supplements may help stave off cataracts and may help thicken bones during the early postmenopausal years and in women who never used estrogen-replacement therapy. Clinical studies suggest that it can fight high blood pressure.

What you'll find: Vitamin C supplements come in 250-, 500-, 1,000-milligram and even higher dosage tablets and capsules as well as powder that you can mix into water or juice.

Whatever form you buy, don't waste your money on natural vitamin C supplements. "There's no difference between synthetic and natural vitamin C—it's exactly the same molecule," says Jeffrey Blumberg, Ph.D., chief of the antioxidants research laboratory at the U.S.D.A. Human Nutrition Research Center on Aging at Tufts University in Boston.

How much to take: The Daily Value is 60 milligrams, an amount researchers now concede is too low to prevent disease. Aim for 200 to 500 milligrams a day, says Dr. Blumberg.

Be aware: Taking more than 1,000 milligrams of vitamin C a day can cause diarrhea in some people. If this happens to you, immediately stop taking vitamin C. If you want to take more than 1,000 milligrams, start with 250 milligrams and increase the dose every few days as your tolerance increases, says Dr. Blumberg.

Vitamin E

What it is: An antioxidant nutrient, vitamin E is found in nuts, seeds, and vegetable oils.

How it delays aging: Research suggests that vitamin E's antioxidant power may help prevent heart disease and cancer, boosts the immune system, and possibly helps normalize blood sugar levels in people with diabetes.

Vitamin E also seems to slow the progression of Alzheimer's disease. Researchers at Columbia University and other centers gave 341 people with moderately severe Alzheimer's disease 2,000 international units (IU) of vitamin E a day for 2 years. At the end of the study, researchers concluded that E had slowed the mental deterioration of those people by about 25 percent, mainly in their ability to perform everyday tasks such as dressing, using the toilet, and eating.

What you'll find: Vitamin E comes in 100-, 200-, or 400-IU capsules. It's also available in liquid.

Recent studies have found that our bodies absorb the natural form of vitamin E (d-alpha tocopherol) more effectively than the synthetic kind (dl-alpha tocopherol). You'll pay more for the natural kind, however.

How much to take: The Daily Value is 30 IU—not enough, suggests some research, to head off heart disease or other illnesses. Aim for 100 to 400 IU, recommends Dr. Blumberg. Take vitamin E with a meal that contains a small amount of fat. You'll absorb it better.

Be aware: If you are taking anticoagulant drugs, use vitamin E only with medical supervision, says Dr. Blumberg.

Aerobics:
The Breath of Life
and Longevity

Air. We can't see it, and we don't think about it. But each of us breathes about 5,000 gallons of the stuff every day, and without it, we'd survive only 8 short minutes.

It's also one of the keys to staying young and healthy.

All day long our muscles and organs get a minimal amount of oxygen as we breathe normally, but if we want to take advantage of oxygen's anti-aging effects, we need to get a little extra. It turns out that the best way to do that is with aerobic exercise. That means huff-and-puff movement, like brisk walking, swimming, biking, and hiking.

When we exercise aerobically, our muscles demand more oxygen and blood than when we're just sitting on the sofa watching television. To fill the demand, our hearts beat faster and stronger, and we start to breathe more heavily.

Cash In on the Benefits

All that huffing and puffing—along with everything else that happens when we exercise—does us a great deal of good. It's like a low-risk investment that yields tremendous short- *and* long-term profits. Here are some of the immediate youth-enhancing benefits exercisers can cash in on.

Boosts metabolism. All that heart-pounding, lung-filling exercise burns a lot of calories and elevates our metabolism, says Miriam E. Nelson, Ph.D., director of the Center for Physical Fitness at Tufts University School of Nutrition Science and Policy in Boston and author of *Strong Women Stay Young.*

As women, we can use all the help we can get. When we hit our thirties, our metabolisms begin to slow by 2 to 5 percent per decade.

Our metabolic rates are already 10 to 12 percent lower than men's. That's partly because pound for pound women have more fat and less muscle than men—and fat burns virtually no calories. Muscles, on the other hand, burn lots of calories as they contract and stretch, making them our metabolism's best buddy.

Why is our metabolism so important? Because it's what helps us control our weight. As it slows, so does our body's ability to use up the calories we eat before they're converted to fat,

Dr. Nelson says. Exercise for at least 30 minutes every day, and you'll maintain or even *lose* weight by giving your metabolism a daily boost.

Boosts energy. Try this the next time you're falling asleep at your desk: Go take a brisk 10- to 15-minute walk. Chances are that you'll feel refreshed and energized when you return. "After it's over, you feel like your energy level is really surging," says John Duncan, Ph.D., an exercise physiologist at Texas Woman's University Center for Research on Women's Health in Denton. A number of things probably go on in your body to create that energy boost, he says. One is that your brain releases feel-good chemicals called endorphins—the same ones that, in excess, create the "runner's high" that marathoners often experience.

Reduces stress. Studies show that exercise is a great stress buster. And the best part is that you don't have to run a 3-minute mile to take that load off your shoulders. Researchers at the University of Georgia in Athens found that anxious college women cut their anxiety in half just by leisurely riding an exercise bike for 20 minutes.

Makes falling asleep E-Zzz. If you've been counting more sheep than a shepherd lately, you're not alone. Women age 40 and older are especially prone to insomnia as they begin to experience the hormonal changes that usher in menopause. Aerobic exercise can improve your sleep by reducing stress, tiring you out, and regulating your body temperature.

The best time to exercise for improved sleep is in the late afternoon, according to Peter Hauri, Ph.D., co-director of the Sleep Disorders Center at the Mayo Clinic in Rochester, Min-

nesota. The body goes through a cycle of rising and falling temperatures throughout the day. When your temperature is at its lowest point, it's easiest for you to fall asleep. Vigorous exercise in the afternoon can boost your body temperature for up to 5 hours, so your temperature will drop just in time for bed.

The worst time to work out is less than 1½ hours before you normally hit the sack, when your body temperature will still be elevated. But everyone is different, adds Dr. Nelson. As long

---

CELLULITE: IS IT INEVITABLE?

Dimples on our cheeks are cute. Dimples on our thighs and butts are not. In fact, cellulite ranks with wrinkles and gray hair as one of the most unwelcome signs of aging.

To get rid of the ripples, women have tried everything from exotic creams to deep massage. But as you might expect, a low-fat diet and regular aerobic exercise turn out to be the most effective therapies. That's because the primary cause of cellulite is weight gain.

When you put on weight, your fat layers expand, but not in a smooth, uniform way, explains Grant J. Anhalt, M.D., acting chief of dermatology at Johns Hopkins University School of Medicine in Baltimore. There are areas where the skin is anchored down by fibrous bands that tunnel through the fat and attach to the muscle. It's those anchors that cause dimpling.

"It's more pronounced in women who are overweight," says Toby Shawe, M.D., assistant professor of dermatology at the Medical College of Pennsylvania–Hahnemann University Hospitals in Philadelphia. "But practically every woman—overweight or not—will get some degree of cellulite," she says.

We can thank our hormones for that. Part of the female hormone estrogen promotes weight gain on the thighs and butt, says Dr. Shawe.

When fat cells take residence on the lower half of the body, they are more likely to get crowded and push against the skin, which creates the bulged and puckered look of cellulite.

As we age, our skin also tends to lose its tautness, especially if we don't exercise. Exercise tones the muscles underneath the skin, which keeps skin taut and eliminates surface lines that can show up on skin stretched by fat. And that can add to the rippling effect.

Genetics play a role as well. "Cellulite is often more noticeable in some people because of heredity," Dr. Anhalt says.

But the years don't have to deposit dimples where they aren't wanted. "The best way to get rid of cellulite is to prevent it," says Jessica Fewkes, M.D., assistant professor of dermatology at Harvard Medical School. "That means starting early with good habits like exercise and a healthy diet."

If the dimples have already developed, you have a few choices. First, you can simply learn to live with them—and still be a very attractive woman. "It's not going to detract from you as a woman unless you let it," Dr. Fewkes says.

Or you can lose those extra pounds and tone your hips, thighs, and buttocks with exercise. Two other options are liposuction, which removes the excess fat, or a mechanical massage called Endermologie, which smooths out the dimples. But either of those will cost you a bundle—from several hundred to several thousand dollars, depending on the procedure. Endermologie averages at $1,400 for a series of treatments.

As for massage and those creams that claim to reduce cellulite: "They don't work," Dr. Anhalt says.

chology at the University of California, San Diego.

Exercise can also make you feel better about your body as you find yourself becoming more fit. The more attractive we feel, the friskier we usually are, he says. And finally, exercise has been found to boost the levels of the hormone responsible for sex drive in men, according to a study done by Dr. Case and colleagues at the University of California, San Diego. And that effect may be similar in women, Dr. Case says.

Eases menstrual cramps. When cramps hit, you're probably not in much of a mood for a jog. But women who exercise regularly experience fewer and less painful menstrual cramps. "We're not sure exactly how exercise helps, but it may be that fit women have tighter abdominal muscles, and that may be beneficial somehow," says Mary Lang Carney, M.D., medical director of the Center for Women's Health at St. Francis Hospital in Evanston, Illinois. Exercise also relaxes us and produces those "happy hormones" called endorphins, which may help relieve the discomfort as well.

Treats you to a natural facial. Ever hear the term *pregnant glow*? Well, exercise can give your face that same rosy radiance. The glow probably occurs after exercise because of the extra blood your heart pumps throughout your body, explains Priscilla Clarkson, Ph.D., professor of exercise science and associate dean of the University of Massachusetts School of Public Health in Amherst. What's more, women who exercise regularly may feel better about themselves. And when you're happier, your face tends to exude that charisma, she says.

as you cool down adequately before tucking yourself in and you don't have problems sleeping, exercising at night is fine.

Revs up your sex drive. If your libido is in low gear, exercise may give it a turbo-boost. Experts say that aerobic exercise can put the sizzle back in your sex life in a number of ways. First, it reduces stress.

When we're more relaxed, we're often more interested in having sex, says David Case, Ph.D., a research specialist in the department of psy-

Disease-Proof Your Body

While the immediate benefits of aerobic exercise may be remarkable, its long-term benefits are even more impressive. Regular exercise increases your vitality, endurance, flexibility, and balance—all things that tend to decline as we age. Fit women not only live longer, they also function as well as unfit people 20 years their junior. But the most significant benefit of exercise is undoubtedly its role in disease prevention. "If you look at a list of all the health problems that occur as you age, exercise has been shown to reduce almost all of them," Dr. Clarkson says. "There's no pill, no medicine that can do that, but exercise can." Here are just some of the conditions exercise can counteract.

Heart disease. Regular aerobic exercise helps prevent heart disease by improving several risk factors: It lowers blood pressure and cholesterol, controls weight, reduces stress, and improves cardiovascular fitness, says Elizabeth Ross, M.D., a cardiologist at Washington Hospital Center in Washington, D.C. The link between exercise and heart health is so strong that even people who already have heart disease can lower their risk of having a heart attack by exercising.

Cancer. Exercisers have a lower risk of developing breast and colon cancer. An 11-year study of more than 1,800 women (average age 75) conducted by James R. Cerhan, M.D., Ph.D., and researchers at the Mayo Clinic in Rochester, Minnesota, found that those who walked, gardened, or did housework several times a week cut their breast cancer risk to half that of inactive women, while those who did more vigorous activity—such as swimming or running—at least once a week were 80 percent less likely to develop breast cancer. And when it comes to colon cancer, in 1996 the Surgeon General's report concluded that physical activity protects against it.

Diabetes. People who exercise regularly have a significantly lower risk of developing Type II diabetes. A 6-year study of more than 8,600 subjects, conducted by researchers at the Cooper Institute for Aerobics Research in Dallas, found that those who were least fit had a four times greater risk of developing diabetes than those who were most fit.

Stroke. Regular exercise can cut your stroke risk in half, according to a recent study conducted by researchers at the Harvard School of Public Health. Swimming 5 hours a week, gardening 6 hours a week, or walking an hour a day for 5 days a week are all ways of dramatically reducing your chances of having a stroke.

Depression. Exercise can help relieve mild depression by raising levels of feel-good substances in the brain and by reducing stress, according to June Primm, Ph.D., a clinical psychologist and associate professor of pediatrics and psychology at the University of Miami School of Medicine. In fact, several studies have shown that aerobic exercise is just as effective as psychotherapy at treating mild depression.

Osteoporosis. Regular exercise can help prevent osteoporosis, the disease that causes women's bones to become so weak that they easily break. A study of nearly 240 postmenopausal women between the ages of 43 and 72 found that those who walked about a mile a day (7.5 miles a week) had denser bones than women who walked less than a mile a week.

Arthritis. At one time doctors told patients with arthritis *not* to exercise. But now we know that exercise—especially walking—can actually ease arthritis pain. A study at Wake Forest University in Winston-Salem, North Carolina, assigned elderly people with arthritis of the knee to do aerobic exercise, strength training, or no exercise. After a year, those who did best were in the aerobic exercise group. They reported less pain and disability than the nonexercise group and were able to walk, climb stairs, and get in and out of the car more easily.

Liven Up Your Lifestyle

Escalators. Leaf blowers. Riding lawn mowers. Self-propelled vacuum cleaners. Remote controls. Power windows.

Little by little we have managed to engineer physical activity out of our lives, says Russell Pate, Ph.D., professor and chairperson of the department of exercise science at the University of South Carolina in Columbia. In fact, a Scottish researcher estimates that people in the United Kingdom burn 800 fewer calories a day compared to 25 years ago.

In the United States, 60 percent of the population incorporates little or no physical activity into their lives. If you're among America's legion of couch potatoes, here's some good news: You don't have to take up tennis or become a marathon runner to enjoy the benefits of exercise. Research shows simply increasing your physical activity provides the same health benefits as a structured exercise program—which is why most experts now recommend trying to work 30 minutes of accumulated moderate activity into your day.

The key word here is *accumulated.* Ten minutes here and there of raking, vacuuming, walking, and playing catch with the kids all adds up. "To make your lifestyle more active, think about what you need to

WOMAN TO WOMAN
She Walked Off the Weight and Feels Years Younger

As she approached the big 4-0, Terri Politi was 25 pounds over-weight—and painfully aware of every extra pound. Her clothes didn't fit right, she felt flabby, and, perhaps worst of all, increasingly sluggish. In other words: Old. Then, 5 months before her birthday, the Sedalia, Missouri, resident, now 41, found the secret to weight loss and peeled off 20 pounds in 4 months. Here's how she turned back the clock.

There I was, hitting one of those big milestones in life, and I was feeling heavier than ever—even heavier than when I was pregnant. I thought, "It's going to be hard enough just to turn 40. I want to do this gracefully." I knew that I could feel better and look better if I just set my mind to it. So in September, I started my quest and gave myself only a few months—by my birthday in January—to reach my goal.

Weight Watchers helped me get a handle on my eating, and that was important, but I wanted to do more. So I began working out with free weights early in the morning, at least three times a week for about 20 minutes each session.

I did start to feel better, yet even that wasn't enough. I decided to start walking on our treadmill for 30 to 35 minutes after every weight workout. I had just enough time to do that, see the kids off to school, jump in the shower, and be at work by 8:00 A.M.

Then, one of my girlfriends at the office and I decided to start a walking program. We have a big church here in town, which had put in a gymnasium, so during lunch break, we went over to check it out. When we found out that 14 times around the gym was a mile, we made it our goal to walk a mile or more three times a week.

Sure enough, by the time January rolled around, I had lost 20 pounds—so I bought myself a little brown dress with a border print along the bottom. I had never owned a simple straight-cut dress before because I always felt my hips were too big to wear something like that. But I like how I look and feel in it.

I have so much energy now and feel so much better about myself that I don't feel like I'm over 40 anymore. I feel as if I'm in my midthirties again.

do each day and how you can make those tasks more physical," Dr. Clarkson suggests. That may mean selling the leaf blower and canning your cleaning lady. Or you can try some of the following lifestyle-makeover tips from our experts.

Turn off the TV. "The first step toward improving your fitness is limiting your sedentary activity," Dr. Nelson says. And one of the most common inactive pastimes is watching TV. Even if you're not a channel-surfing TV junkie, you probably turn on the set at least a few times a week. Try to cut back by 1 hour every week until you've managed to trim an hour of sitcoms, soaps, or game shows from each day. You'll be surprised at how much time you'll have on your hands.

If you can't bear to miss an episode of *NYPD Blue*, then put a piece of exercise equipment—like a treadmill or stationary bike—in front of the tube and turn your TV time into a workout, suggests Dr. Ross.

Walk and talk. If you have a cordless telephone, take advantage of your wireless freedom. Walk around the house or up and down the stairs while chatting on the phone. You'll catch up with your friends while you catch a short workout.

Dodge the drive-through. More and more service businesses are installing drive-up windows for our convenience: banks, fast-food restaurants, even drugstores and photo developers. "As we take on these conveniences, we don't realize how much they decrease the amount of physical activity in our daily lives," Dr. Clarkson says. So resist the quick convenience of the drive-up window and walk into the bank to make your transaction.

Pick the farthest spot. When it comes to your health, the best parking spot is not the one that's closest. Park a few blocks away, and you can work in a quick walk, Dr. Pate says.

Take the stairs. Make a conscious effort to use the stairs instead of an elevator or escalator, Dr. Pate says. It may not seem that significant, but think about how often you'd opt for stairs. Every day? Once a week? A few times a month? No matter what, it can really add up.

Eliminate e-mail. If you send e-mail to coworkers who are in the next office or just down the hall, consider taking an e-mail vacation. Deliver the message in person, and you'll save yourself from gaining 11 pounds over a decade. That's how much weight a Stanford University researcher calculated you would gain if you spent 2 minutes an hour sending e-mails to coworkers instead of walking down the hall to speak to them.

Pay the pound a visit. Getting a dog may help get you off your duff. Pups make great walking partners—and they don't let you off the hook easily when a walk may not be what you had in mind.

Plant a garden. Playing in the dirt was fun when we were kids. And now that we're grown-ups, we can make more than mud pies. Whether you grow flowers, herbs, or vegetables, you'll burn almost as many calories as taking a moderate aerobics class—plus you'll connect with the earth, says Dr. Nelson.

12 Tips for a Better Workout

Fitness is a step-by-step progression, Dr. Nelson says. If you're already fairly active—or you've recently succeeded in adding more physical activity to your lifestyle—the next step to getting fit is simple: Whatever you're doing now, do *more*.

This is where aerobic exercise comes in. But don't worry. You still don't have to join a health club or take an aerobics class (unless you want to). The great thing about aerobic exercise is that there are so many different activities to choose from—dancing, biking, swimming, playing tennis. The list goes on and on.

No matter which activities you choose, you'll get the most out of your workout if you follow these practical pointers.

Put on your dancing shoes. If you're dancing, that is. And running shoes if you're running. Walking shoes if you're walking. You get the idea. "As we get older, our feet, ankles, shins, and knees are more vulnerable," says Joan Price, certified fitness instructor, speaker, and writer from Sebastopol, California, and author of *Joan Price Says, Yes, You Can Get in Shape!* "Wearing the right shoes for your activity can protect you by cushioning and stabilizing your feet and basically serving as mini-shock-absorbers."

Seek out support. When you work out, make sure that you wear an appropriate sports bra that holds your breasts close to your body, Dr. Nelson suggests. Otherwise, all the movement that's involved in aerobic exercise can start your breasts sagging southward. "It amazes me that a lot of women don't wear a sports bra when they exercise," she says. "When you don't, the repeated movement will actually stretch the breast tissue and make it less elastic."

Warm up. Your car isn't the only thing that needs to be warmed up before all its parts are lubricated and ready to roll—you have your own engine and parts that need to run a few minutes before shifting into high gear. "A warmup provides a gradual transition from rest to the physiologic demands of exercise," Dr. Pate says. Basically, a good warmup gets your blood pumping, limbers up your ligaments and tendons, and loosens your muscles so that you reduce your risk of injury.

Light stretching and a slow version of the activity you're about to do work best, Dr. Pate says. Walk more slowly before you pick up the pace, for example, or swing the racket and hit a few

balls before playing a round of tennis. You could even march or jog in place—anything that gets your arms and legs moving for 5 minutes.

Cool down and stretch. Your body needs to downshift its gears slowly, rather than going from brisk walking to a sudden halt. The cooldown is similar to the warmup, only instead of gradually picking up the pace, you gradually slow it down. This lowers your heart rate gradually so that you don't feel dizzy or faint, Dr. Nelson explains.

After your workout is also the best time to stretch because your muscles are still warm. A good 20- to 30-second stretch of each of the major muscle groups—that's your arms, legs, abdomen, back, and rear end—helps to build flexibility and prevent injury.

Beat blisters. Whether you walk, jog, hike, or hit the tennis courts, a bad case of blisters can put the brakes on your physical activity fast. To prevent blisters before they start, cover your clean, dry feet with your regular antiperspirant, suggests lead researcher Joseph Knapick, Sc.D., at the U.S. Army Center for Health Promotion and Preventative Medicine in Aberdeen Proving Ground, Maryland.

You can use any kind—spray, stick, or roll-on. Just make sure to hit every nook and cranny of your feet. Try it every day for 5 days before your run or hike, or use it once or twice a week indefinitely. It works by reducing sweat, which creates the friction that causes blisters. And it helped 80 percent of U.S. Army cadets stay blister-free after a 13-mile hike.

One note of caution: If you develop a rash or experience any skin irritation, try using the antiperspirant every other day or switch brands. If the irritation continues, stop using it.

Drink up. When you exercise, you sweat out more fluids than you would just sitting on the couch. And since your muscles are about 70 percent water, you need to replenish those fluids so that you don't start to feel weak before your workout's over. A good rule of thumb is to drink an 8-ounce glass of water before and after you exercise and to have half a cup every 15 to 20 minutes during your workout, says Felicia Busch, R.D., a nutritionist in St. Paul, Minnesota, and a spokesperson for the American Dietetic Association.

Leave your worries behind. To get the relaxation benefit of exercise, you have to wind down while you're working out. We already mentioned a study conducted at the University of Georgia in Athens where stressed-out college students cut their anxiety in half by riding exercise bikes for 20 minutes. Simply taking time out from daily worries may have been responsible for the drop in anxiety, the study authors say, because another group of women who studied while riding still had high anxiety levels afterward.

Add weights to firm flab. Many experts recommend combining your aerobic exercise with strength training. Why? Because together they give your flab a one-two punch. "Aerobic exercise burns fat while strength training tones muscle," Dr. Nelson says. And the result is a firmer, shapelier body.

What's more, strength training gives your metabolism an extra boost by building muscle, which burns more calories.

And the stronger your muscles are, the more you'll get out of your aerobic workout. "You'll be able to exercise longer, and you won't feel as tired afterward," Dr. Nelson says.

Slow down the music. The aim isn't to add romance to your workout, but to keep the music at a comfortable pace, especially if you're participating in an aerobics class that requires fancy footwork or using a step. "The music should be slow enough for you to put your foot all the way down," Price says. "Staying on your toes because the music is too fast puts you at risk to injure

your foot or leg." If you feel uncomfortable asking the instructor to use slower music, or if you're using a workout video and can't change the music's speed, then do the move at half-speed, she suggests.

Make it fun. When we were kids, exercise was a ball. We sprinted up the stairs, we ran home for dinner, we jumped when we heard something exciting, and we looked forward to recess. "Exercise should still be playtime," Dr. Ross says. "Most women have so many responsibilities in addition to their jobs that if exercise becomes just one more thing on our 'must do' list, we won't stick with it. That's why I encourage women to find something that's fun. Put the kids in a stroller and the dog on a leash and go for a walk. Dance with your husband for 15 minutes before you sit down to eat. Take the kids roller-skating or ice-skating. Or go for a bike ride."

Grab a partner. Even if you're not square dancing, a partner can help you out in several ways. First, she can motivate you when you're feeling tired or discouraged, Dr. Nelson says. Second, exercising with a friend can turn your workout into a social activity—so it's more fun. And most important, a friend can help you stay committed. If you don't feel like exercising but your friend is counting on you, you're more likely to put on those sneakers and hit the road.

Stick with it. Cardiovascular fitness requires maintenance. If you work out 5 days a week for several weeks, for example, and then cut back to exercising just 1 day a week, you'll lose 90 percent of your gains in 12 weeks, Dr. Duncan says. So do yourself—and your heart—a favor and make exercise a permanent part of your routine.

Weather Your Workout

Many women use their workouts as a way to take in some scenery. But exercising outdoors brings with it comfort and safety issues. These simple tips will help you weather your workout so that you can enjoy your time in the great outdoors.

Save your skin. Always apply sunscreen to any part of your body that's exposed. This simple habit will help prevent wrinkling and skin cancer, says Grant Anhalt, M.D., acting chief of dermatology at Johns Hopkins University School of Medicine in Baltimore. Wear a sunscreen with a sun protection factor (SPF) of 15 if you're out in the morning or late afternoon. But switch to an SPF of 30 to 45 if you're out between 10:00 A.M. and 2:00 P.M. for substantial periods of time—like if you're shooting 18 holes, fishing, or boating, he says.

Shade your eyes. Eye doctors at Johns Hopkins University School of Medicine polled more than 2,500 people on their history of sun exposure. Those who had been in the sun the most had a 57 percent greater likelihood of having a cataract. The best way to protect your peepers is to wear sunglasses or clear prescription glasses and a wide-brimmed hat whenever you exercise outdoors—even in the winter when snow causes sun glare, says Dr. Pate.

Follow the dress code. If you bike, walk, or jog during the day, wear bright colors so that drivers can easily spot you. If you work out at night, dawn, or dusk, outfit yourself with some type of reflective gear so that you can be seen from

WOMEN ASK WHY

Both of my knees are the same age, so why is one causing me all kinds of trouble when I exercise?

While both of your knees are the same age, they aren't always subject to the same punishment. Do you favor one hand over another when you write, drive, or toss a ball? Chances are good that you've battered one of your knees more often when walking, jumping—or even falling—over the years.

That cumulative punishment is called microdamage. But as we get older, it can cause big problems. Like a dried-out rubber band, our connective tissues simply become less flexible, making them more prone to tearing.

So how can you avoid knee pain during—or after—you exercise? For one thing, you need to start slowly. Our bodies do change and adapt to our workouts, but not if we try too much all at once. The key is to increase your activity and intensity gradually over time.

If you do begin to experience some pain—whether it's in a knee, ankle, or some other joint—that's your body's way of telling you that you need to slow down. If your pain is minor and goes away in a day or so, you probably won't have to stop exercising, but proceed with caution.

If your pain persists or is severe, you'll need some rest and treatment. One of the most common therapies for knee or ankle pain is called RICE—an acronym that stands for rest, ice, compression (wrapping with a bandage), and elevation. When using ice in a pack or bag, make sure to cover it with a thin towel to protect the skin. If you don't feel better after 2 or 3 days' rest, you may need to see a doctor.

Expert consulted
Russell Pate, Ph.D.
Professor and chairperson of the department
*   of exercise science*
University of South Carolina
Columbia

the front and rear. And make sure to sport bright or reflective clothes on rainy and foggy days, too.

Layer it on. If you weather winter workouts, make sure to put on several layers of clothing. That way you can shed layers as needed so that you don't overheat. It may feel frigid outside, but your body temperature will rise as you exercise, and you may get hot, Dr. Duncan explains.

If it's really cold, experts suggest wearing three layers. Use fabrics such as Coolmax, polypropylene, or ThermaStat blends as an inner layer to wick moisture away from the skin. As a middle layer, insulate by trapping a layer of warm air next to your body with fleece, wool, or Bipolar fabric. The outer layer should shield you from weather extremes. Gore-Tex, fleece, and wind jackets and pants are all good outer protectors.

Outsmart hay fever. If you find yourself sneezing and rubbing your eyes during allergy season, avoid exercising in the morning or move your workout indoors, suggests Carol Wiggins, M.D., clinical instructor of allergy and immunology at Emory University in Atlanta. During fall and spring hay-fever seasons, the pollen count is highest between the hours of 5:00 and 8:00 A.M. and lowest at night.

Slather after laps. Whether you swim indoors or out, slather on a moisturizer after finishing those laps. Swimming washes away the natural lipids in your skin, making it dry and itchy, says Dr. Anhalt. The best time to moisturize is right after getting out of the pool when your skin is still wet. Doing so helps seal in the moisture that's still on your skin. Moisturizing immediately after getting out of the shower will help to further prevent dry skin.

Water: The Fountain of Youth

The Spanish explorer Juan Ponce de León sailed halfway across the world looking for the fountain of youth. He never found it. You or I, on the other hand, can make it appear instantly by turning on the kitchen tap.

Sound like magic? Not really. Today we know something that Ponce de León didn't: The power of that fountain lies in simple, fresh, clean water.

Your body needs water for all the basic processes of life, which include everything from transporting nutrients to regulating internal temperature. But drinking plenty of water—at least eight 8-ounce glasses a day—can give you benefits above and beyond the basics. It can also help you maintain healthy, younger-looking skin and prevent certain diseases and conditions that can make you feel far older than your years.

Water Down Wrinkles

Nature makes the lesson obvious: Dry out a grape, you get a raisin. Dry out a plum, you get a prune. Wrinkles, wrinkles, wrinkles.

On the other hand, if you're ironing out the wrinkles from a cotton shirt, you moisten it with steam. And if you want to keep roses from wilting, you put them in a vase with water.

So it is with skin. If you want to keep it smooth, supple, and radiant, water is one of the secrets you're looking for. "Healthy skin is about 10 to 20 percent water," says Diana Bihova, M.D., a dermatologist in New York City and coauthor of *Beauty from the Inside Out*. If your skin loses more than half its moisture, it becomes dry and flaky. Even fine lines become more pronounced. Over time, dry skin can age more quickly.

One way to fight back is by using moisturizers. When you moisturize your skin, it plumps up and looks smoother, and fine lines seem to disappear.

The problem is that time makes the going tougher. Our skin gets drier as we get older. Around age 30, oil and sweat glands slow their production and skin is less able to retain moisture, says Dr. Bihova. And as we get closer to menopause and our estrogen levels drop, our skin may dry out even more.

CAN THE COLA TO SAVE YOUR BONES

For many of us who are watching our waistlines, no two words in the English language look so appealing side by side as "diet" and "soda." Unfortunately, what delights the tongue may destroy the bones.

"If you drink four or more cans of cola a day, you are putting yourself at risk for developing osteoporosis even earlier than menopause," says Elizabeth Lee Vliet, M.D., medical director of HER Place Women's Centers in Tucson, Arizona, and Dallas–Fort Worth.

That's because cola soft drinks—both regular and diet—pull calcium from your body in several ways. First, they contain high amounts of phosphorus. When this mineral builds up in your body, it can interfere with the absorption of calcium and slow down your body's natural bone remodeling, says Dr. Vliet.

Second, cola beverages are very acidic. Your body neutralizes the acid by pulling bicarbonate and calcium from your bones.

Finally, the caffeine in cola hinders the kidneys from using calcium properly. As a result, the calcium is lost through urination before it can be absorbed by the body.

And there's yet another problem with drinking soda: If you're slurping half a dozen cans a day, you're probably not drinking any calcium-rich milk. A better bone-saving strategy is to cut back on cola and make sure to get enough calcium through diet and supplements, says Dr. Vliet.

pruny by the last plate, bathing or showering in steamy-hot water may send you hankering for hand-and-body lotion hours later. That's because hot water can dry out your skin. To save face, try soaking or showering in lukewarm water instead of hot.

Switch your soap. Washing with harsh soaps can leave your skin feeling like sandpaper—so stick to gentle cleansers like Cetaphil. They cleanse your skin without irritation and leave behind a moisturizing film. Buy cleansers with ingredients such as water, glycerin, sodium lauryl sulfate, cetyl alcohol, and stearyl alcohol.

Time it right. The best time to moisturize is right after a shower or bath, when your skin is still wet and the moisture can be sealed in.

Water the air. Dry winter air wicks moisture away from your skin, leaving it dull and dry. But running a humidifier adds moisture to the air and prevents water loss through your pores.

Drink to Your Health

Water not only lubricates your skin, it keeps everything inside your body flowing smoothly as well. "Most people are minimally dehydrated, and that can impact practically everything a person does," says Felicia Busch, R.D., a nutritionist in St. Paul, Minnesota, and a spokesperson for the American Dietetic Association. You can lose 1 to 2 percent of your body weight in water without ever feeling thirsty. And once you have lost that much water, your body can't function at its best. You start to feel tired,

That's where water comes in. Drinking plenty of water is important. Whether you sip it or soak in it, water moisturizes your skin. But that's not all you need to do. "Drinking an ocean of water is not, by itself, going to repair your dry skin," says Dr. Bihova. And simply slathering on lotion won't end your dry skin dilemma either. Here, Dr. Bihova shares some secrets to getting the most from moisture.

Keep your cool. Just as washing a sinkful of dishes in hot water leaves your hands dry and unfocused, weaker, and slower. You may even get a headache—all things that make you feel sluggish and older than you really are.

A well-watered body has what it needs to stay young and healthy. Here are some ways you can use water to help you feel your best.

Keep your colon healthy. Drinking the standard eight glasses a day may lower your risk for colon cancer. Researchers have found that women who drink more than five glasses of water a day have about half the risk of colon cancer as those who drink two or fewer glasses.

Stay regular. Older people are five times more likely to be constipated than younger folks. And chronic constipation can lead to uncomfortable and painful conditions like hemorrhoids or diverticulitis.

To keep your bottom end feeling as young as a baby's bum, drink up. Having enough water in your pipes can help prevent and relieve constipation, especially if you eat a high-fiber diet. That's because water softens your stools so that they can move more easily through your system.

Slim down. Drinking lots of water keeps you trim—first, by helping you burn fat more efficiently. And second, if you drink it right before meals, it fills you up, so you eat less.

Beat bladder infections. Almost half of the 16,000 women surveyed by *Prevention* magazine and the American Medical Women's Association a few years ago had experienced a bladder infection and had tried drinking plenty of water

to treat it. Eight out of 10 said it worked for them. Doctors say that all those fluids may help by flushing infection-causing bacteria out of your system.

Stave off kidney stones. When you don't drink enough water, wastes that are normally dissolved and removed in your urine may become concentrated in crystals, which could lump together to form a kidney stone.

LIFE EXTENDER
Green Tea: The Longer-Life Elixir

Trading in your coffeepot for a tea kettle could add years to your life. Research shows that drinking green tea may offer you a slew of benefits, from helping to lower your cholesterol and blood pressure to reducing your risk of heart attack and stroke. This Chinese pot of gold also helps protect the immune system, aids digestion, and prevents cavities and gingivitis. But someday we may find that green tea's most impressive life-extending benefit comes from cancer-fighting antioxidants called polyphenols.

Animal studies show that substances in green tea may protect against several types of cancer, including tumors of the skin, breast, stomach, colon, liver, lung, and pancreas. Studies on humans are less clear but suggest that drinking green tea may lower the risk of getting certain cancers such as stomach, colorectal, and pancreatic. A study of more than 35,000 middle-aged women in Iowa found that those who drank at least 2 cups of black, green, or oolong tea a day significantly reduced their risks of getting digestive tract and urinary tract cancers.

What's more, a study found that women with early-stage breast cancer who were regular green tea drinkers had a better prognosis than those who weren't. Green tea drinkers also develop cancers much later in life. In one study done in Japan, women cancer patients who had consumed more than 10 cups of green tea a day developed the disease an average of 8.7 years later than those who drank fewer than 3 cups a day.

Prevent muscle soreness. When you're physically active—whether you're doing work around the house, gardening, or playing tennis—water can ward off the day-after aches that make you feel all washed up. If you're slightly dehydrated, your body taps the water that's stored in your muscles. That can decrease your strength and increase your risk of micro-scopic muscle damage, which shows up as soreness the next day, says Scott Hasson, Ed.D., chairperson of the department of physical therapy at the University of Connecticut in Storrs.

A good rule of thumb is to drink a glass of water before and after physical activity as well as a half-cup every 15 to 20 minutes during the activity, he says.

A Female Disadvantage

Your body's about 50 percent water, so think of yourself as a glass that's half full. To keep that level from dropping, you have to drink at least eight 8-ounce glasses of water a day. Staying hydrated is especially important for women because their bodies store less water than men's, says Busch. That's because women have less muscle, which holds a lot of water, and more fat, which doesn't. As a result, a woman's well runs dry more quickly than a man's, so you have to be more faithful about replenishing what you lose each day. Women who are pregnant or nursing need to drink even more water, Busch adds—at least 10 to 12 glasses a day.

Still others need extra water to keep their skin supple and their bodies working at their best. Here's how to know if you are getting your fill.

Check the conditions. You need to drink more than the average eight glasses a day if you're sick, if you live in a hot climate, if you spend a lot of time inside heated or air-conditioned buildings, if you do a lot of public speaking (like a teacher), or if you're larger than average, Busch says.

Drink before you're thirsty. You can't use thirst to determine when you need to fill up, because you can lose as much as 5 percent of your body's water supply before feeling thirsty, Busch says. To prevent this, try water breaks: when you first wake up, when you get to the office, at break times, before meals, and before bed. One glass of water at each of these times will keep you well-hydrated on regular days.

As you get older, your sensitivity to thirst decreases, so it becomes even more important to drink throughout the day, whether you're thirsty or not, adds Joanne Curran-Celentano, Ph.D., associate professor of nutritional sciences at the University of New Hampshire in Durham.

Clear things up. Check the color of your urine. "It should be almost clear, a pale yellow," says Lucia Kaiser, R.D., Ph.D., a nutrition specialist at the University of California, Davis. If it's not, you need to drink more fluids.

Ways to Fill Your Tank

If downing 2 quarts of water a day sounds like more than you can stomach, don't dry-dock just yet. These tips from our experts will help you get a handle on staying hydrated.

Call in a substitute. All eight glasses don't have to be water. Other beverages like milk, juice, seltzer, and sparkling water can also count toward your daily intake. So can foods that contain lots of water such as soups and juicy fruits such as watermelon, cantaloupe, grapes, and oranges. But don't count beverages that contain alcohol or caffeine; they actually cause you to lose more water than you take in.

Punch up the flavor. If water's too plain for you, try flavored water or squeeze in fresh fruit like lemon, lime, orange, or pineapple. Or toss frozen-juice ice cubes into your water—they add flavor as they melt. For soft-drink fans who miss the carbonation, try adding sparkling water to $\frac{1}{4}$ cup of juice.

Sip before you snack. People often think that they're hungry when they're actually thirsty. So have a drink first; it may take care of your hunger pang.

Measure it out. Fill a 64-ounce pitcher and try to empty it by the end of the day.

Keep it close. Have a glass or bottle of water with you when you're at your desk, outdoors, in your car, or at the gym.

Take it slow. Sipping rather than gulping will prevent you from feeling bloated.

Make a pit stop. Every time you pass a water fountain, take a drink.

PART TWO

Keeping Up Appearances

Erasing the Lines of Time

There are many milestones in a woman's life: The beginning of her monthly cycles. The day of her wedding. The birth of her first child. The day she spots her first wrinkle . . .

Oh, mirror, mirror on the wall, why does it have to happen? We know we accumulate wisdom with the years, but must we also accumulate wrinkles? The sight of those tiny crinkles under our eyes or the first faint creases along our foreheads (not to mention the appearance of broken capillaries and age spots), can make us want to turn away from our own reflections (or, like the evil queen in *Snow White*, just smash the mirror).

Faced, so to speak, with less-than-youthful skin, we have two choices. We can accept it and make friends with our frown lines. Or we can fight it every step of the way.

Want to arm yourself for battle? We have considerable control over how our skin ages and plenty of ways to keep it glowing and youthfully smooth, ways that don't include weird facial exercises, skin creams with hundred-dollar price tags, or trips to a plastic surgeon's office.

Even if you haven't yet spied that first wrinkle, you still have good reason to lavish your still-youthful skin with TLC. "The earlier you start to care for your skin, the bigger the difference you'll see as you age," says Francesca J. Fusco, M.D., a dermatologist in New York City.

To achieve more youthful-looking skin, it's important to understand how it changes through the years—and why.

Why Skin Gives In

Obviously, aging alone takes its toll. Our skin's protective outside layer, the epidermis, becomes thinner and increasingly fragile. Oil glands produce less oil, leaving the skin drier and more sensitive. The number of blood vessels decreases, so you lose the rosy glow of youth. Moreover, aging slows down the speed at which you replace old cells with fresh, new ones.

Genetics, too, plays a role in how skin ages. Fair-skinned women, for example, show signs of premature aging faster than women with darker skin. That's because fair skin contains less melanin, the substance that gives skin its pigment and helps protect it from the sun, explains Linda K. Franks, M.D., a dermatologist in New York City.

DON'T NEGLECT YOUR NECK

No matter how young you may look from the chin up, if you don't lavish some care on your neck, your age will be an easy read. Like the skin around our eyes, neck skin is a prime age-revealer. "It's thinner than facial skin, with practically no oil glands, so it's extremely vulnerable to dryness and sun damage," says Jennifer Ridge, M.D., a dermatologist in Middletown, Ohio.

To prevent further damage, start using these save-your-neck strategies now.

Pamper your throat. It's not necessary to use special neck creams, says Dr. Ridge. Simply lavish your neck with the same gentle cleanser and rich moisturizer you use on your face. Apply the moisturizer with firm upward strokes.

Take the Teflon approach. Coat your neck daily with a sunscreen, moisturizer, or makeup foundation that has a sun protection factor (SPF) of at least 15. If you are using sunscreen alone, use a chickpea-size dollop.

Apply sunscreen to your chest, too. "Open collars and scoop-neck dresses expose your chest to the sun," says Dr. Ridge.

To further protect your neck, keep a small tube of sunscreen in your handbag and apply it several times a day—every 2 hours if you're out in intense sun. Why? Because a single application in the morning won't protect your neck all day. "Sunscreen sweats off, it rubs off—in a few hours, it's gone," says Dr. Ridge.

Protect while you sleep. When we sleep on a pillow, we tend to squash our chins against our necks, says Dr. Ridge. Over the years, as our skin loses its ability to snap back into place, these "sleep wrinkles" on our necks will become permanent.

To keep your neck smoother, trade in your regular pillow for a neck roll, suggests Dr. Ridge. These small, log-shaped pillows, available in medical supply stores and catalogs, are designed to keep your chin and neck in alignment. They also keep your neck skin taut. Be warned, however: Neck rolls can have an unfortunate side effect. "You may snore more," says Dr. Ridge, "but your neck will look better."

Defy nature. To reduce the wrinkles on your neck, use lotions or creams containing glycolic acid, one member of a group of substances known as alpha hydroxy acids (AHAs), says Dr. Ridge. These natural fruit and milk acids chemically slough off, or exfoliate, the buildup of dead cells on the surface of your skin, exposing the newer, fresher skin underneath.

You'll find products containing AHAs, most of which use glycolic acid, in the skin-care aisle of any drugstore. Look for brands that contain 10 percent glycolic acid. To get the most dramatic results, however, you may need a stronger concentration—up to 25 percent—for which you'll have to see a dermatologist.

A dermatologist may also suggest tretinoin (Retin-A or Renova). Like glycolic acid, these products chemically exfoliate the skin's top layer. They also penetrate its second layer, the dermis, where they help form collagen, the fibrous material that gives skin its youthful plumpness. Although they both work well, says Dr. Ridge, Retin-A and Renova are both prescription drugs, so you can only get them under a doctor's supervision.

But that's only part of it. No matter how many candles may decorate your birthday cake or how fair your complexion is, to a large extent, your skin's "age" depends on how well you take care of it.

The cardinal skin sins are basking in the sun and smoking cigarettes. Both speed the breakdown of collagen and elastin, the structural proteins that give skin its youthful plumpness and

OUT, DAMNED SPOTS

Freckles on kids' faces? Cute. Freckles on *our* faces? Unless we were blessed with them at birth, not cute at all.

"If you're 35 or 40 and have 'freckles' in areas that you never did as a kid, your skin has sustained sun damage," says Jennifer Ridge, M.D., a dermatologist in Middletown, Ohio.

What we commonly call freckles actually fall into two categories, she explains. True freckles, or ephelides, are the little brown spots we're born with. They're simply spots of melanin, the substance that gives skin its pigment. We inherit them from our parents; those of us with light skin and hair are more likely to have them. While true freckles come out in the sun, they also tend to disappear as we age.

Like true freckles, false freckles, or solar lentigines, are made of melanin. But unlike inherited freckles, lentigines sprout for a specific reason: They are the skin's attempt to defend itself from the sun. And they don't fade with the years. They get worse.

While lentigines aren't dangerous, they do mean we've sustained sun damage, which makes skin more vulnerable to sun-induced skin cancers, says Dr. Ridge. The antidote to future sun damage? Sunscreen. Coat your face and neck with a product that has a sun protection factor (SPF) of at least 15. Or use moisturizers and makeup with SPF 15 sunscreen.

---

ability to snap back. The result is premature sagging, wrinkles, roughness, age spots, and blotches.

Other skin agers include chronic emotional stress, poor nutrition, excessive dieting, and drinking alcohol, says Debra Jaliman, M.D., a dermatologist in New York City.

Skin Enemy Number One: The Sun

Ask dermatologists to name the most treacherous skin villain of all, and the sun wins hands down. Sun damage, or photoaging, gives skin the texture of leather and can leave a formerly peaches-and-cream complexion riddled with wrinkles, spots, blotches, and broken blood vessels.

How can something that feels so good on our bare skin wreak so much destruction? In a word: radiation.

The sun gives off two types of ultraviolet (UV) radiation: UVA, sometimes called tanning rays, and UVB, the so-called burning rays. Until recently, UVA rays were thought to be harmless. In fact, UVA light is still used in tanning beds. But dermatologists now know that both UVA and UVB rays are equally destructive to the skin. Over the years, these rays slowly but steadily break down collagen and elastin, until one fine day—presto! You've entered the Face-Lift Zone.

The damage starts earlier than you may think. "Eighty percent of the sun damage takes place before the age of 20," says Rhoda S. Narins, M.D., clinical associate professor of dermatology at New York University Medical Center and a dermatologist in New York City and White Plains, New York.

Most vulnerable to photoaging are women with fair skin and light hair and eyes, and women who have grown up in high altitudes, where UV rays are at their most intense, says Dr. Franks. "I see women in their twenties who have grown up in Colorado or skiers who have spent years in high-intensity sun, and they already have fine lines and wrinkles under their eyes."

Think your darker skin is immune to solar assault? Think again, says Dr. Franks. Even African-Americans and olive-skinned people of Mediterranean ancestry, whose skin contains more melanin than that of lighter-skinned people, can sustain sun damage. "I've seen many olive-skinned women who have extremely sun-damaged skin," she says. "They seem to develop sunspots, or so-called liver spots, earlier."

Sunscreen to the Rescue

Wouldn't it be great if there was a miracle product that could protect skin from the sun's assault? That could actually *prevent* sun-induced wrinkles?

There is. It's called sunscreen.

Think of sunscreen as Armor All for your skin. No matter what your age, slathering on sunscreen *right now* can help prevent future sun damage, say dermatologists.

It may also fend off the formation of wrinkles. "It takes years of sun exposure to make wrinkles, but the skin is damaged before wrinkles actually appear," says Dr. Franks. "By using sunscreen now and turning off the ongoing assault, you can delay or even prevent wrinkles."

There are two types of sunscreens. Physical blocks, the first type, contain zinc oxide or titanium dioxide and act as a force field, literally blocking UVA and UVB rays from reaching the skin. Zinc oxide—that pasty white stuff lifeguards used to slather on their lips and noses—is the more powerful of the two.

Thankfully, it's now possible to reap the benefits of zinc oxide without looking as though you just came from a Halloween party. Nowadays, most nonprescription physical blocks, which are

WOMEN ASK WHY

Why does my skin look so awful when I don't get enough sleep?

The baggy eyes, dark circles, puffiness, and sallowness your skin manifests after a bout of insomnia or an all-nighter happen for the same reason people with jet lag look lousy: Your body clock—and your hormones—are out of whack.

Most people's body clocks are set to let them sleep at night and wake them up in the morning. These internal clocks are also programmed to release certain hormones at certain times of the day.

You may have noticed that at night, before you go to bed, your eyes are swollen and you look tired and puffy. Why don't you look that way in the morning? Assuming that you have had adequate sleep the night before, your hormones rebound for the morning ahead and "prepare" your skin to wake up.

One hormone that peaks primarily in the morning is cortisol, which is secreted by the adrenal glands. Cortisol has a dramatic impact on skin: It aids in regulating swelling. With changes in the levels of cortisol, swelling can go up or go down.

When you get enough sleep, cortisol peaks on schedule—in the morning. It helps reduce morning puffiness and contributes to your skin's looking rested and refreshed. On the other hand, a late night or a bout of insomnia throws off your body clock, so cortisol doesn't peak when it is supposed to. You arise with a pale, puffy face.

Expert consulted
Andrew Pollack, M.D.
Chief of dermatology
Chestnut Hill Hospital
Philadelphia

available at a dermatologist's office, contain zinc oxide that has been micronized (that is, crushed into virtually invisible particles). You can also check on the Internet for these products, since they aren't commonly available in stores.

Chemical sunscreens, the second type, contain specific chemicals that absorb both UVA and UVB rays. Avobenzone, also known as Parsol 1789, is one of the most widely used and most effective chemical sunscreens, notes Dr. Franks.

But using sunscreen alone can't keep the sun from aging your skin if you insist on starting—and finishing—the latest 300-page bestseller while you bake on the beach. "Even the best sunscreens allow some UV rays to penetrate the skin," says Dr. Fusco.

A Sunscreen Primer

So now you're convinced that the sun turns skin to toast? You've sworn to use sunscreen every day? Great. Now all you have to do is choose the right product and use it correctly. Here's how.

Follow the numbers. For everyday protection, use a sunscreen that contains a sun protection factor (SPF) of at least 15, says Dr. Franks, and apply it 30 minutes before going out into the sun. Every day. Even when you don't see a hint of sun. (Clouds can block brightness, but they may allow as much as 80 percent of UV light to reach your skin.)

If you plan to spend time on the golf course, tennis court, or ski slope, use a sunscreen with an SPF of 30, says Dr. Fusco. Ditto, if you spend a lot of time on a boat or at the beach. Sun reflects off water and bounces onto your skin, which intensifies its damage. And since perspiration, excessive toweling, and water can wash sunscreen away, reapply it occasionally. You may want to try one of the many waterproof sunscreens available, but remember that it also has to be reapplied.

Broaden your protection. A sunscreen's SPF factor measures only its UVB coverage, says Dr. Franks. So make sure that the sunscreen you buy is labeled "broad-spectrum," meaning that it absorbs both UVB and UVA rays. Most broad-spectrum sunscreens contain Parsol 1789 or titanium dioxide.

Don't be stingy. Use a marble-size amount of sunscreen to cover your face, two "marbles" to cover your neck and chest, says Dr. Fusco. If you

---

GLOW FOR IT—WITHOUT THE SUN

To get a sun-kissed glow minus the wrinkles, try a self-tanning lotion, says Mary Ronnow, a paramedical aesthetician (skin-care specialist working in a doctor's office) at Northern Nevada Plastic Surgery in Reno. Unlike the "bottled tans" of the past, the new generation of sunless tanners is less likely to streak—and, better yet, won't turn you the color of a carrot.

The active ingredient in self-tanners, dihydroxyacetone (DHA), interacts with the amino acids in your skin's top layer, turning skin darker in the process. This "tan" fades within a few days, as your skin sheds dead cells.

To get the best bottled tan possible, follow this step-by-step plan from Ronnow.

Shower, then rinse well. Self-tanners "take" better when they are applied to skin free of body oils, perspiration, and cleanser residue.

Slough off roughness. While you're in the shower, exfoliate with a loofah, body mitt, or exfoliating cleanser to remove dry skin and rough patches. Smooth skin absorbs DHA more evenly, so your tan won't look splotchy.

Moisturize. To smooth skin even more, slather on your favorite body lotion. Let it penetrate until you can no longer see or feel it on your skin.

Take it from the top. Apply a self-tanner thinly and evenly, from face to feet. Use a dime-size amount on your face, another to cover your neck, but don't apply tanner on the eyelids or into the eyebrow. Blend down your chin and into your neckline. To tan the backs of your hands, put a dollop of self-tanner on a cotton ball, then wipe across the backs of your hands and fingers. Don't use too much tanner around your hairline or on knees, elbows, and ankles; these areas seem to "grab" more DHA and can become especially dark.

If you're using a spray-on tanner, spray the product lightly and evenly on one body part at a time. Then blend quickly, following the guidelines above. To apply to your face, spray the product on your hand and blend evenly and well.

Whatever product you choose, don't use it in a hot, steamy bathroom. The heat will turn it runny, making it difficult to apply.

Tan-proof your palms. When you're finished, immediately scrub your hands with a loofah or a product with scrubbing grains. Get between your fingers, too.

Keep glowing. Reapply a sunless tanner a second time the same day until you're as dark as you want to be. To maintain your tan, reapply it every few days.

One caution: Self-tanners won't protect your skin from the sun. So choose a brand that contains a sunscreen with a sun protection factor (SPF) of 15 or above. Two that do are Bain de Soleil and Physician's Formula. You can also apply sunscreen over your new "tan" to get the same protection.

use makeup or moisturizer and a sunscreen, apply the sunscreen first. You want it as close to your skin as possible.

Use "built-in" sunscreens. To save time, money, and medicine-cabinet space, use a moisturizer or foundation with an SPF of at least 15. "For everyday use, these products are as effective as sunscreen alone, when used properly," says Dr. Fusco. "But you must remember to apply the equivalent of 1 teaspoon of foundation to assure the sun protection factor promised."

Wrinkle-proof your kisser. Sun damage can eventually crinkle lips, too. So wear a lipstick or lip balm with added sunscreen to help keep lips soft and youthful looking, says Dr. Fusco.

Skin Tips for Sun Junkies

Ask any dermatologist, and she'll tell you to stay out of the sun between 10:00 A.M. and 4:00 P.M., when the sun's rays are strongest. While that's sound advice, we're women, not vampires. Some of us live in sunny climates, some of us spend weekends in our gardens, and others love to golf or play tennis. If you must bask, follow the tips below. They will help to "super-boost" your sun protection.

Use your head to save your skin. While in intense sun, wear a hat with a brim that's at least 4 inches wide (think: a Mae West–size chapeau). Forget the sailor hats and baseball caps; neither offers much protection from full-bore sun, says Dr. Jaliman.

Take a cue from Foster Grant. Wear wraparound sunglasses designed to block 95 to 100 percent of UVA and UVB rays, says Dr. Jaliman. Why wraparounds? They will protect your eyes from harmful UV rays while completely blocking the crow's-foot zone.

Be slightly shady. While out in intense sun, periodically retreat to a shady spot, says Dr. Jaliman. At the beach, park yourself under a big umbrella. Also, while on hikes or on the water, if it's not too hot out, wear tightly woven clothing. It will help keep UV rays from penetrating your skin. But if you'll fry, wear at least a hat, sunglasses, and plenty of sunscreen.

Clean Up Your Act

When dentists say that good oral hygiene protects your teeth and gums, you know exactly what they mean. Extending the metaphor, practicing good *skin* hygiene can help protect skin from premature wrinkling. The tips below can help you clean up youth-stealing skin habits.

Don't be a smoke face. Here's another good reason to quit. Current smokers are two to three times more likely to develop premature wrinkling than nonsmokers, according to research conducted at the University of California, San Francisco. That's because smoking causes the fibers of the skin to lose their elasticity sooner and become more susceptible to wrinkling. It also literally strangles skin. The nicotine in cigarettes narrows blood vessels, preventing oxygen-rich blood from reaching the tiny capillaries in the top layers of the skin. This oxygen deprivation makes skin dull, gray, and leathery—a condition so well-known that it has a name: smoker's face.

The good news is that smokers will see an improvement in the appearance of their skin in just 60 smoke-free days, says Dr. Franks, the time it takes for skin to replace itself twice.

Get enough Zzzs. As obvious as it sounds, try to sleep at least 8 hours a night. "Like any other organ, your skin needs time to repair itself, and sleeping is excellent downtime," says Dr. Franks.

Sleep on your back. If you can't, learn. Scrunching your face into your pillow for 30 to 40 years will eventually press wrinkles into your skin, says Dr. Jaliman.

The Perfect Cleanser

The skin-care industry spends millions trying to convince us that their products hold the secret to smooth, line-free skin. Dermatologists say, "Bah!"

"I'm a big fan of simple, basic skin care," says Dr. Franks. "All you need is a gentle cleanser and a moisturizer." The mini-guide below can steer you toward cleansers that work best for *your* skin.

As mentioned earlier, the skin's oil glands produce less oil as we age. The right cleanser washes away dirt and makeup but leaves oil where it belongs—on your face.

If you're dry, go creamy. "The drier your skin, the more gentle your cleanser should be," says Dr. Fusco. She suggests Oil of Olay Foaming Face Wash or Cetaphil. Cetaphil is a soap-free cleanser that's free of skin-irritating fragrances, additives, and preservatives.

Dissolve away oil. Oily skin tends to be thick, so it can tolerate a stronger cleanser. Try an oil-binding liquid cleanser formulated for oily skin, such as Neutrogena Oil-Free Acne Wash, a cleanser with salicylic acid. If you prefer a bar cleanser, try Neutrogena Oily Skin Formula Facial Cleansing Bar, suggests Dr. Fusco. Or try a gel cleanser formulated for oily skin.

If you're sensitive, pick a kinder, gentler cleanser. Try Cetaphil, says Dr. Fusco. Dermatologists often recommend this product for people with sensitive skin. If not, pick a cleanser such as Almay that's labeled hypoallergenic, meaning that it contains fewer ingredients than regular products and few or none of the ingredients known to cause allergic reactions.

Cleanse correctly. The way you cleanse your skin is just as important as the product you use, says Dr. Fusco. Here's the correct way to wash your face. If you're using a liquid, lotion, or gel cleanser, place about a teaspoon of cleanser in the palm of your hand. Massage it gently into your skin using the balls of your fingers. Rinse your face with warm water until all the cleanser is removed (about five or six times) or wipe off the cleanser with a soft, damp washcloth. If you're using a bar cleanser, hold it under water to wet it, then work up a lather in the palm of your hand. Using the balls of your fingers, massage your face in a circular motion for 30 seconds, then rinse, as above. Pat skin dry—never rub it.

Avoid scrubbing grains or pads. "Prolonged exfoliation can actually make the skin become drier and accent fine lines," says Dr. Fusco. Enough said.

Navigating the Moisturizer Maze

Moisturizers are like diet books—there's a new one on the market every day. But don't be seduced by high-priced, high-tech products: All a moisturizer can do, says Dr. Fusco, is soften skin and moisturize. It cannot erase lines.

If you're dry, oil up. The drier your skin, the more hydrating elements your moisturizer should contain, says Dr. Fusco. So pick a product formulated with ingredients such as glycerin, hyaluronic acid, or dimethicone. Eucerin and Moisturel are two of many good choices, she says. They slow down natural moisture loss throughout the day and prevent further skin dehydration.

Or go the natural route. "Olive oil is a great moisturizer," says Dr. Jaliman. Of course, it's not for someone who is acne-prone, and it's best used as a before-bed treatment because olive oil can't protect your skin from the sun. (Plus, you'll smell like a Greek salad while you're at work.)

If you're oily, go light. Oily skin may feel dry, the result of harsh cleansing products formulated with ingredients such as alcohol that strip away the skin's natural oils, says Dr. Fusco. Try a moisturizer that contains humectants (ingredients that attract and hold water), such as glycerin and sodium PCA, she says. These ingredients trap water in your skin with no greasy shine. Also, choose a lotion. Lotions are lighter than creams and tend to contain less oil, so they won't clog pores.

If you're sensitive, think basic. Use a hypoallergenic moisturizer, says Dr. Fusco. Apply it to a test area first to see if you tolerate it well. Pure glycerin (available at drugstores) or petroleum jelly can be effective, she adds, but you should avoid them if you're acne-prone.

Consider eye creams. It's fine to use your regular moisturizer around your eyes. But if you have sensitive skin or your eyes are easily irritated, consider buying moisturizing eye cream, says Dr. Fusco. Creams made to be used specifically around the eyes are less likely to aggravate delicate undereye skin—or your peepers themselves.

The Care and Feeding of Youthful Skin

Years ago, we thought that chocolate and french fries could cause zits. Much too late, we found that it wasn't true. What *is* true: Consuming a *healthy* diet shows on the face. To feed your skin young, read on.

Quench your skin. The Great Water/Skin Debate has raged since your own mother was a girl. But according to Dr. Franks, "Drink, drink, drink—eight glasses a day, at least." Drink more during the winter, when the indoor air is dry. "Skin continually loses moisture to the air, so it draws on the reserve of water that's in the skin's deeper layers.

Back off the booze. Alcohol dilates blood vessels. In some women, consuming more than moderate amounts of alcohol will cause their vessels to continually dilate and constrict, stretching them like rubber bands until they have no more snap, says Dr. Franks. Eventually, vessels just stay dilated, she says, leading to spider veins and broken capillaries.

Alcohol also causes the skin to lose water, "and dehydrated skin is more sensitive to sun damage," says Dr. Franks.

Eat your skin vitamins. Consume a mother lode of fruits and vegetables rich in the antioxidant nutrients vitamin C, vitamin E, and beta-carotene, says Dr. Fusco. Antioxidants help protect skin from the damaging effects of free radicals, unstable oxygen molecules that are generated after exposure to the sun.

Strawberries, papaya, kiwifruit, navel oranges, and sweet red peppers are especially rich sources of vitamin C. Vitamin E can be found in cooking oil, wheat germ, nuts, and seeds. Spinach and other dark green leafy vegetables, along with deep orange fruits and vegetables such as carrots, sweet potatoes, cantaloupe, and pumpkin, are bursting with beta-carotene.

Take extra C. Consider taking extra vitamin C, which the skin needs to build collagen, says Dr. Jaliman. She suggests 1,000 milligrams of vitamin C a day. You can choose a multivitamin that contains this amount or consume a separate vitamin C supplement.

Say no-no to yo-yo dieting. Avoid gaining and losing weight over and over. "It leads to wear and tear on collagen and elastin," says Dr. Jaliman. Steer clear of starvation diets, too. Very low calorie diets deprive your skin of the nutrients it needs to thrive, she says.

Special Problems of Aging Skin

As if coping with laugh lines and crow's-feet wasn't enough, we also have to deal with other age-related skin problems, from puffy eyes to large pores. But take heart. Here's what experts suggest you can do on your own to brighten, tighten, or just plain hide these bothersome flaws.

To shrink puffy eyes: Believe it or not, some women use the hemorrhoid product Preparation H. This product contains hydrocortisone, a topical steroid that reduces inflammation, says Dr. Jaliman. Does it really send eye bags packing? "My clients say it does," she says, "but the tightening effect is temporary." Be warned that long-term use can thin the skin and lead to acne, premature wrinkling, and broken blood vessels. Consult your physician before using this product around your eyes.

OUR EYES AT 30, 40, 50

According to Jennifer Ridge, M.D., a dermatologist in Middletown, Ohio, here is a general idea of what your face can expect as time marches on.

In our thirties: We may get dark circles under our eyes, as the skin under our eyes thins and exposes the pigment beneath. We may also notice our first lines or wrinkles. They may be barely noticeable or quite prominent, depending on whether we have dark or light skin and how much sunlight we were exposed to in our teens and twenties. In some of us, the fat pad under our cheeks (the malar fat pad) begins to droop, pulling the skin under our eyes with them.

In our forties: Our skin begins to lose its youthful plumpness and elasticity, and we may see our first lines and wrinkles. We also develop deeper lines at the corners of our eyes. These crow's-feet, as they're called, are especially prominent if we have fair skin, if we've smoked, or if we were sun junkies in our youth.

In our fifties: Wrinkles become deeper, especially in the crow's-foot zone. Sagging becomes more prominent, causing our upper lids to droop toward our lash line.

If daubing hemorrhoid cream under your eyes sounds less than appealing, reduce eye baggage with more conventional tactics, says Dr. Jaliman. Sleep with your head elevated so that fluid doesn't pool under your eyes. Reduce your intake of salt, which encourages fluid retention. Or keep a stash of teaspoons in the freezer and place them over your eyes when you wake up with puffs. The cold metal will reduce the swelling.

To erase dark circles: Use an over-the-counter fading cream (such as Porcelana) that contains a 2 percent concentration of hydroquinone, suggests Dr. Jaliman. Circles should lighten in 1 to 2 months. This product also fades age spots. (To conceal dark circles with makeup, see page 70.)

To brighten sallow skin: Ask a dermatologist about glycolic acid, suggests Sheryl Clark, M.D., a dermatologist in New York City. This alpha hydroxy acid (AHA), derived from sugarcane, removes dead, complexion-dulling cells from the skin's top layer, revealing the new, fresh skin beneath. And you can see results in as little as 2 weeks. You can obtain glycolic acid through your dermatologist. Over-the-counter formulations often are too low in concentration to be effective.

To hide spider veins or broken capillaries: These fine red lines that squiggle across the cheeks or nose can be removed with either a laser or an electric needle, says Dr. Jaliman. It's easier just to conceal them with makeup.

To minimize large pores: Use pore-cleansing strips, like Bioré or Pond's, on your nose, forehead, chin, or cheeks, suggests Dr. Fusco. "Dirt dilates pores," she says. "If they're not all plugged up with gunk, they'll look smaller." While these products are safe and effective, don't use them more than once every 2 weeks.

Astringents and clay masks can also temporarily minimize pores, says Dr. Fusco. The skin temporarily plumps up, which makes pores appear smaller. Use this trick only on special occasions, however. "Overuse of these products can leave skin tight, dry, and flaky," she says.

To discourage frown lines: Place a piece of waterproof cloth tape across your forehead before bed, suggests Dr. Jaliman. "The tape will keep you from frowning in your sleep, which will prevent some wrinkling." Tape won't prevent crow's-feet, however. "You don't scrunch your eyes when you sleep," she says.

Cosmetic Nutrients: Bottled Youth

Let's face it: We're bedazzled by so-called anti-aging products that promise smoother, more youthful skin. But do these lotions and potions, so temptingly packaged (and often, so astronomically priced), actually work?

That depends on how you define *work*.

Some over-the-counter anti-aging products contain specific ingredients that can help skin look better temporarily, says Debra Price, M.D., clinical assistant professor in the department of dermatology at the University of Miami. The first ingredient is glycolic acid, a member of a group of fruit acids called alpha hydroxy acids (AHAs). The second is topical vitamin C—more specifically, L-ascorbic acid, a particular form of vitamin C.

If your skin appears dull and has lost its glow, an over-the-counter glycolic acid product may make it appear smoother and fresher, says Dr. Price. And when teamed with sunscreen, vitamin C gives skin extra protection against sun damage, the primary cause of wrinkles, roughness, age spots, and discoloration.

But the weak concentrations in over-the-counter products cannot—repeat, *cannot*—permanently alter the skin. So while they may exfoliate and smooth your skin, they won't erase wrinkles. "If they could, they would be classified as drugs, and they wouldn't be available at the cosmetics counter," says Dr. Price.

There is one substance that research shows *can* permanently alter the structure of skin: tretinoin, a derivative of vitamin A and the active ingredient in Retin-A and Renova. These products are drugs, so they're only available with a doctor's prescription. But they are the way to go if you want to reduce fine wrinkles and crinkles, roughness, or pigment changes such as age spots, says Nia Terezakis, M.D., clinical professor of dermatology at Tulane University School of Medicine in New Orleans.

Still, we know how irresistible those tiny jars, bottles, and perky cosmetics-counter salespeople can be. This guide to the hottest anti-aging skin products will tell you how they work, how to use them, what they can (and can't) do, and whether to buy them over-the-counter or from a dermatologist or skin-care salon.

Get Glowing with Glycolic Acid

Derived from sugarcane, glycolic acid is the most common AHA in over-the-counter anti-aging products. It's also the most effective, says Sheryl Clark, M.D., a dermatologist in New York City.

Research has shown that the chemicals in glycolic acid slough off, or exfoliate, the buildup of dead cells on the skin's top layer. "Removing these dead cells makes skin look smoother and gives it a glow," says Francesca J. Fusco, M.D., a dermatologist in New York City.

The average drugstore glycolic acid product costs around $10. But expect to pay $20 or more—sometimes much more—for the ritzier glycolic acid products offered by major cosmetics companies.

At the cosmetics counter. Most over-the-counter glycolic acid products contain less than 10 percent glycolic acid. These low concentrations won't do a thing for lines and wrinkles, say experts. But some women who use these products like the way they make their skin look smoother and fresher.

Research suggests that at concentrations of 10 percent or higher, glycolic acid may stimulate the formation of collagen, the connective tissue in the skin's second layer (the dermis) that gives skin its youthful plumpness and strength. A few over-the-counter products, such as the Alpha-Hydrox and Aqua Glycolic lines, do contain 10 percent glycolic acid.

Glycolic acid products are easy to use. Once a day, you simply apply two to three pea-size

"BETA" THAN ALPHA HYDROXYS?

If your skin stings and burns when you use products containing glycolic acid, which is an alpha hydroxy acid (AHA), try a kinder, gentler wrinkle fighter: salicylic acid, also known as beta hydroxy acid (BHA).

Found naturally in the bark of willow and sweet birch trees, salicylic acid works at much lower concentrations than glycolic acid, says Albert M. Kligman, M.D., emeritus professor of dermatology at the University of Pennsylvania School of Medicine in Philadelphia. That means that it causes less redness, stinging, and burning.

In one study involving hundreds of women, those who used salicylic acid on their faces reported much less irritation than the group who used glycolic acid.

Apparently, their skin looked better, too. A panel of 30 judges who looked at before-and-after photos concluded that the salicylic acid group showed more improvement in their skin than the glycolic acid group. The judges specifically looked at fine lines, blotches, and abnormal pigmentation of the skin.

Those of us who battle breakouts along with wrinkles may also want to use salicylic acid, says Dr. Kligman. Like glycolic acid, salicylic acid sloughs off, or exfoliates, the top layer of skin. It also penetrates into our pores, liberating the trapped dirt and oil that lead to acne. That's why it's the active ingredient in many over-the-counter acne medications.

Anti-aging products formulated with BHA can be found in your local drugstore. Three examples are Oil of Olay's Daily Renewal Cream with Beta Hydroxy Complex, Almay's Time-Off Revitalizer Daily Solution, and Aveda's Exfoliant.

amounts to the clean, dry skin of your face and neck, says Dr. Clark.

At the dermatologist's office. If you're sporting a few faint lines, consider seeing a dermatologist, who can offer a variety of products that can contain up to 25 percent glycolic acid. "It's clear that higher concentrations of glycolic acid—12 percent and above—are more likely to benefit aging skin," says Dr. Price. Expect to pay from $10 to $60, depending on the product line and how much glycolic acid it contains.

The advantage of going to a dermatologist is that she can examine your skin and recommend the concentration of glycolic acid that's right for you. If you have dry or sensitive skin, she may recommend using a product formulated with 8 percent glycolic acid, says Dr. Clark. Then in a month or so, after your skin adjusts, she may jump you to a higher percentage.

Oily skin can tolerate higher concentrations of glycolic acid, she says. So a dermatologist may recommend, right off the bat, a gel or oil-free cream that contains 10 to 20 percent glycolic acid.

You use doctor's-office glycolic acid products the same way as the over-the-counter variety, says Dr. Clark. You're likely to see a noticeable difference in your skin tone within 2 weeks of the first application.

If these products are going to minimize fine lines, expect to wait at least 3 months, says Nicholas V. Perricone, M.D., associate clinical professor of dermatology at the Yale University School of Medicine.

Glycolic Acid: A User's Guide

For your skin to reap the full benefits of a glycolic acid product, it must be used correctly, says Dr. Clark. Here's how to choose and use these products, whether you get them from the corner drugstore or a dermatologist.

Test the waters. Try an over-the-counter product before consulting a dermatologist, suggests Dr. Price. You may find that using a lower percentage of glycolic acid will give you the results you want.

Get the right formulation for your skin. Both over-the-counter and dermatologist's-office glycolic acid products come in creams, gels, and liquids (sometimes called serums). Generally speaking, people with dry skin prefer cream formulations, while those with thicker, oilier skin prefer the gels or the serums, says Dr. Perricone.

Test before you treat. Using glycolic acid isn't without its drawbacks: It can cause some people's skin to sting, itch, or, in rare cases, break out in a rash. So take a skin-sensitivity test before using glycolic acid for the first time, says Dr. Clark. Rub a small amount of the product on the inside of your elbow every day for a week. If there's no redness or irritation in this time, chances are that the glycolic acid won't overly irritate the skin on your face, she says. If you do experience irritation, Dr. Clark suggests that you try using the product only every other or every third day. If that doesn't work, try a lower concentration.

Apply it at night. After you apply glycolic acid, it takes at least 15 minutes for it to penetrate the skin. So if you have only minutes to spend on your morning skin-care routine, smooth on your product before bed, suggests Dr. Clark. Applying moisturizer or makeup immediately after glycolic acid can reduce its effectiveness, she says. Be sure to avoid getting glycolic acid products in or around your eyes.

Use sunscreen. The use of glycolic acid products can make skin more sensitive to the sun than it was before. So without fail, apply a sunscreen with a sun protection factor (SPF) of at least 15 before going out for the day, says Dr. Fusco. Or use one of the many moisturizers or foundations that contain SPF 15 sunscreen.

Quit if your skin cries "ouch!" Stop using glycolic acid *immediately* if your skin becomes intensely red, irritated, or inflamed, says Dr. Clark. While such severe reactions are rare, they do occur, especially in women with sensitive skin.

The "A" Team: Retin-A and Renova

When the acne medication Retin-A was introduced in 1969, women with severe acne cheered. But in 1988, when a study showed that it could also tackle wrinkles, women everywhere stampeded to the nearest dermatologist.

As we mentioned, the active ingredient in Retin-A (and its spinoff, Renova) is tretinoin. While dermatologists still prescribe Retin-A for acne, they also routinely prescribe it for aging skin. Renova is formulated specifically for the treatment of aging skin.

Like glycolic acid, Retin-A and Renova loosen and remove dead cells on the skin's top layer, making it appear smoother. But research also shows that tretinoin increases the skin's levels of collagen, lightens sun-induced freckles and age spots, and improves skin discoloration.

At the cosmetics counter. Since Retin-A and Renova are drugs, you won't find them at the cosmetics counter. What you *will* find, however, are anti-aging products that contain retinol, another derivative of vitamin A, says Dr. Terezakis.

While retinol sounds like Retin-A, there is no conclusive evidence that it *works* like it. As an antioxidant, however, retinol may offer skin some protection from free radicals, those unstable oxygen molecules that are unleashed by sunlight, smoke, and pollution and that may prematurely age skin, explains Dr. Clark.

At the dermatologist's office. Retin-A comes in cream, gel, or liquid formulations and in varying concentrations of tretinoin. For de-wrinkling, most dermatologists prescribe the cream. Renova contains 0.05 percent tretinoin in a cream base.

WOMEN ASK WHY

Why do those anti-aging creams cost so darn much?

There's no *good* reason that purchasing a good skin-care product should require a woman to take out a personal loan. No product on this earth warrants a $70 or $100—or, in some cases, a $300—price tag.

Still, cosmetics companies have their reasons for jacking up the prices of these anti-aging formulations. First, they have to pay big bucks to package and advertise them. A fancy box and a beautiful glass container often cost more than the product they contain. Second, women are willing to pay high prices to look younger, and manufacturers are happy to accommodate on that account.

Unfortunately, many women still believe that the higher the price, the higher the quality. The fact is that lots of $10 products are just as good as more expensive ones, and it's unlikely that any formulation priced over $25 is worth the money.

That said, some *ingredients* in over-the-counter products can, in theory, help aging skin look better. These include antioxidants, like vitamin C and vitamin E, which fight free-radical damage, and substances such as hyuralonic acid and mucopolysaccharides, which help skin hold on to moisture. Products containing alpha hydroxy acid (AHA) can help by exfoliating the skin.

But even if these products do work—and there is no hard proof that they do get rid of wrinkles—they still can't perform miracles. If you're looking for a "miracle" skin-care product, buy a bottle of sunscreen.

Expert consulted
Paula Begoun
Bestselling author
Professional makeup artist
Owner of a small chain of cosmetic stores
Author of Don't Go to the Cosmetics Counter without Me

Whether a dermatologist prescribes Retin-A or Renova depends on skin type. "People with oily skin tend to use Retin-A, while those with dry or sensitive skin prefer Renova because it has the consistency of a really heavy night cream," says Dr. Clark.

Using either one is a no-brainer. Dr. Clark recommends applying two pea-size drops—enough to cover the whole face and neck—to clean, dry skin, either every night or every other night before bed. Dot the medication on each cheek, your forehead, and your chin. Then rub it into your skin, avoiding your upper eyelids. A 2-month supply of either medication costs about $30.

Many people using Retin-A or Renova notice that their skin feels smoother after a month of treatment, says Debra Jaliman, M.D., a dermatologist in New York City. Research shows that the most significant improvement occurs over 4 to 10 months. And the more damaged your skin, the more improvement you're likely to see.

Using Retin-A or Renova does have a downside. Both, particularly Retin-A, can cause skin to swell, burn, itch, or peel. These side effects normally fade in a few weeks as skin becomes used to the medication. But if the irritation continues, a dermatologist may advise applying the drugs less often, or—in the case of Retin-A—prescribe a lower dosage, says Dr. Perricone.

Using Retin-A and Renova

Retin-A and Renova are *drugs*. So don't apply more than indicated, and don't use them more frequently than your dermatologist recommends. Also, don't use Retin-A or Renova if you are pregnant. To get the most anti-aging bang for your buck, follow the tips below.

Start now. Retin-A and Renova seem to prevent wrinkles more effectively than they erase them. So fill your first prescription before you spy the first crinkle, advises Dr. Fusco. "If you're

35 or 40 and have never worn sunscreen or have a history of burning and tanning, don't wait for the damage to show," she says.

Slather on sun protection. Every single day, apply a sunscreen with an SPF of at least 15 or use an SPF 15 moisturizer or foundation, says Dr. Fusco. Because Retin-A and Renova return the skin to its more youthful plumpness, the newer, fresher skin underneath is vulnerable to sun damage.

Soothe irritation right. To reduce temporary redness, flakiness, and irritation, use a hypoallergenic moisturizer with no added fragrances or preservatives, such as Eucerin or Complex 15, suggests Dr. Clark. Or smooth on a dab of over-the-counter hydrocortisone cream every other day.

Also, consider taking 800 international units (IU) of vitamin E a day. Preliminary studies suggest that vitamin E may reduce the irritating effects of Retin-A and Renova, says Dr. Clark. But be sure to check with your doctor before using amounts higher than 200 IU.

Practice kinder, gentler skin care. While using Retin-A or Renova, avoid using astringents or toners with a high alcohol content, products with scrubbing grains, and clay facial masks. Stay out of saunas and steam rooms, too. Since moisture and heat increase blood flow, they also increase the penetration of medications, which can cause redness. All can further irritate skin, says Dr. Clark.

Double the benefits. Ask your dermatologist about teaming Retin-A or Renova with glycolic acid, suggests Dr. Clark. "When they're used together, both seem to be more effective," she says. Generally, you apply the glycolic acid in the morning and the Retin-A or Renova before bed.

Vitamin C: Future Youth?

Topical vitamin C is the Next Big Thing in anti-aging skin care, according to Dr. Clark. Tiny vials of vitamin C "serums" sell at cosmetics counters for $65 and up, and still we empty cosmetics-counter shelves.

Research suggests that topical C can help protect our skin in several ways, says Dr. Price. "There is definitive evidence that topical vitamin C functions as an antioxidant, thereby helping to protect skin against free-radical damage," she says. "There's also strong evidence that it helps protect skin exposed to the sun: When vitamin C is applied to skin, it gets less burned. And topical C may have a protective effect when used in conjunction with sunscreen."

Sounds good so far. But does it "regenerate collagen," "renew elasticity and firmness," and "promote a smoother, firmer, more youthful-looking complexion," as its major manufacturers claim?

According to preliminary research (much of which, by the way, was conducted by folks who are selling the stuff), L-ascorbic acid can, indeed, promote the formation of collagen. Moreover, some dermatologists, including Dr. Clark, swear that the skin of their patients who use topical C appears fresher, more evenly pigmented, less blemish-prone, and, in some cases, less furrowed.

Other dermatologists say the jury's still out on topical C's crinkle-fighting capacity. "There's little scientific data to suggest that topical C definitely reverses wrinkles and promotes the production of collagen, although it may," says Dr. Price.

What does she tell her patients about C? "I tell them that, at this

WOMAN TO WOMAN
She Wanted to Revitalize Her Skin

Just past her 40th birthday, Diane McCurdy, a licensed aesthetician from Philadelphia, received an unwelcome "gift"—her first fine lines and wrinkles. But she didn't get blue. Instead, she started applying a pea-size amount of one of the new "youth" creams to the fair, freckled skin of her face and neck. Did it work? Here's her story.

I was 41 when I noticed that my skin was looking, well, older. I have my father's Irish skin—fair, freckled, very dry. My skin looked dull, felt parched, and I was seeing my first lines.

I had heard that Renova, a prescription cream that gets rid of fine lines and age spots, was really helpful. I happen to work for a dermatologist and asked him if it would work for me. He examined my skin and prescribed Renova.

I've used this thick, virtually fragrance-free cream for 2 years now, and I couldn't be more pleased. My skin looks brighter and rosier. Its texture is much smoother, and the fine lines around my eyes and the vertical lines above my lips are less noticeable.

The difference in my skin has actually made my makeup look better. If you have any lines in your face at all, you know how foundation and powder can kind of cake into them. Renova sloughs off dead cells from the skin's top layer, so your makeup goes on more smoothly.

Looking younger on the outside has improved my inside. My self-esteem is higher. I have more self-confidence—I feel good about myself.

Renova has definitely helped my skin look younger. But I have to credit my sunscreen habit, too. You absolutely have to use sunscreen. Every single day I use a sunscreen with a sun protection factor (SPF) of 20 that contains zinc oxide or titanium dioxide because it gives a much broader range of protection against ultraviolet A and B rays.

A lot of my friends and acquaintances have noticed the improvement in my skin. My husband's reaction? He got his own prescription for Renova. He has Irish skin, too.

point in time, the best way to protect their skin is to use a broad-spectrum sunscreen that contains transparent zinc oxide. And then, if they can afford to, they should use topical C, because the combination will probably be more protective than sunscreen alone."

Typically, topical C is applied to clean, dry skin once a day. According to the manufacturers of Cellex-C, one of the most popular topical vitamin C products, fine lines will become less noticeable in 3 to 8 months.

Don't Get Lost at "C"

Keep in mind that topical C has not been conclusively proven to reduce wrinkles. ("With topical C going for $70 a pop, I'd put my money on tretinoin," says Dr. Terezakis.) On the other hand, if you want to maximize the effectiveness of your sunscreen, it may be worth buying—if you can afford it. Here's what to look for.

At the cosmetics counter. With some notable exceptions, vitamin C creams are unlikely to work, says Dr. Price. Mostly because vitamin C is extremely unstable and loses its potency rapidly, explains Dr. Clark. There's also no telling how much vitamin C these products contain—or if it's in a form that won't break down as soon as you open the jar or that has already been broken down by other ingredients.

The *only* topical C products that have been scientifically tested for their effects on aging skin contain a 5- to 15-percent concentration of L-ascorbic acid, a specific form of vitamin C. They also have a low (acidic) pH, which helps the skin absorb the vitamin. They're pure formulations that don't contain extra ingredients, such as sunscreen or other vitamins, and they are kept airtight in their dispensers to prevent oxygen from breaking down the vitamin C and turning it brown. These products have been shown to penetrate the skin and protect against free-radical formation.

Currently, several brands of topical vitamin C meet these standards, say Dr. Price and Dr. Clark. And you can find them all in the cosmetics departments of fine department stores, licensed skin-care professionals' offices, and skin-care salons. You can also get them through mail order.

Cellex-C's High-Potency Serum contains 10 percent L-ascorbic acid. Another brand, EmerginC, offers a serum (with 12 percent L-ascorbic acid) and a cream (with 10 percent). The Skinceuticals line features a High-Potency Serum 15 (with 15 percent L-ascorbic acid) and a High-Potency Serum (with 10 percent).

Getting the Most from C

Want to see for yourself whether topical C smooths away your fine lines and wrinkles? To increase your chance for success, follow the expert-recommended tips below.

Store C correctly. To prevent vitamin C cream or serum from breaking down too quickly, store it in a cool, dark place, says Dr. Clark. It's okay if the cream turns honey-colored or amber, she says. But if it turns dark brown or begins to smell funny, toss it.

Use a pump formula. A pump bottle seals out oxygen, which will extend the life of the product, says Dr. Clark.

Use C before Zzzs. It takes a full hour for L-ascorbic acid to properly penetrate the skin, says Dr. Clark. So rather than use a topical vitamin C product in the morning—and waiting to apply your moisturizer and makeup—apply it at night, before bed. If you're also using Retin-A or Renova, or other alternate products, then apply topical C on your "off" nights, she says.

Keep the sunscreen flowing. While topical C seems to offer skin extra protection from the sun, it is *not* a sunscreen, says Dr. Price. So keep slathering on that SPF 15.

Makeup That Enhances

There comes a time in almost every woman's life when, standing bleary-eyed in front of her bathroom mirror, she offers up a brief prayer of thanks:

Thank God for makeup.

Using cosmetics is the simplest way to minimize or conceal age-related skin imperfections—instantly. Foundation softens the appearance of fine lines, brightens skin, and hides discoloration. Concealer erases dark circles under your eyes or broken capillaries on your cheeks. Blusher returns the bloom of youth to a tired-looking complexion, while lipstick gives pale or sallow skin a welcome jolt of color. A touch of powder ensures that makeup lasts longer and colors stay truer.

What's more, makeup has gone high-tech. Today's products are lighter and sheerer. One-shade-fits-all makeups are a thing of the past, and there's a wide selection of cosmetics formulated specifically for dry and aging skin.

If you wear little or no makeup, you may be afraid that starting now will make people think you've developed a sudden interest in a career with Barnum and Bailey. But rest assured, you'll look just terrific. According to Laura Geller, makeup artist and owner of Laura Geller Make-Up Studios in New York City, makeup is virtually goof-proof once you learn the three golden rules: Less makeup is more. Don't be afraid of color, just use it subtly. And blend, blend, blend. Be sure to blend your makeup carefully, particularly in the zones shown in the illustration.

To put your best face forward, try some of these suggestions made by Geller and other makeup artists who are experts at enhancing youthfulness in mature skin.

Foundation: Add Color, Subtract Flaws

Mature skin needs color *and* subtle concealment. The right foundation delivers both. And no one will know you're wearing it but you.

Most flattering formulation: Before choosing a foundation, answer these two questions: How much do you need to hide? And does your skin need more moisture or less?

Foundations come in three weights, or amounts of coverage: sheer, medium, and full. Generally speaking, mature skin is most flattered by a sheer- or medium-weight foundation, says Doreen Milek, director of the Studio Makeup Academy, a school that trains professional makeup artists, in Hollywood, California. "A sheer foundation may not cover blotches or discoloration, while full-coverage foundations, which are meant to cover birthmarks or other serious skin flaws, can look cakey and chalky."

Foundations also come in two basic formulas: oil and water. Oil-based foundations, such as Maybelline Revitalizing Liquid Make-Up with SPF 10 Sunscreen, Almay Time-Off Age-Smoothing Makeup, or L'Oréal Visible Lift Line-Minimizing Makeup,

ARE YOU A MAKEUP ABUSER?

Makeup can help us erase the years—unless we don't apply it correctly. Then it can actually *add* them, says Doreen Milek, director of the Studio Makeup Academy, which trains professional makeup artists, in Hollywood, California. Check the list below to see if you're making these common makeup goof-ups.

Wearing too much makeup. Some of us try to hide the years beneath layers of cosmetics, says Paula Mayer, a makeup artist in San Diego. "The truth is, using too much makeup makes you look older." If your blusher looks more like windburn than a subtle wash of color, if you use a very thick foundation and apply it with a heavy hand, or if your eye makeup reminds you of Cleopatra's, chances are you're looking older than you have to.

Not blending in. Too many of us end our foundation at our jawlines, or don't blend our blusher into our foundation. That's the Tammy Faye Bakker approach to makeup—and it adds years, says Milek. So blend your foundation, blusher, and eye shadow until you can't see where they begin and end.

Wearing those "Groucho" eyebrows. Okay, you don't make your eyebrows *that* dark and heavy, but you get the picture. "Use a powder eye shadow on brows," recommends Mayer. "It gives brows a soft, natural look that brow pencils can't." She uses a deep gray shadow on brunettes and women with gray hair, and a soft brown on blondes and redheads.

Using too much liner under eyes. "It makes eyes look smaller," says Laura Geller, makeup artist and owner of Laura Geller Make-Up Studios in New York City.

Being stuck in the past. We wouldn't be caught dead in the miniskirts we bought in 1968 or the gaucho pants we loved in 1978. But many of us think nothing of applying makeup the same way we did when the Supremes (or Led Zeppelin) broke up.

The point: Makeup styles change, and to look more youthful, we have to keep up. "Not adapting your makeup to reflect the times is aging," says Milek. "Your face has changed, and your makeup should reflect those changes."

Here are some of the ways—subtle and not-so-subtle—that makeup styles have evolved over the years.

1960s

1970s

1980s

1990s

are best for dry or mature skin, says Geller. Oil-based foundations add moisture to skin, giving it a dewy appearance.

Whatever foundation you choose, select a product that contains added sunscreen, says Milek. It will help fortify your skin against sun damage.

Can't-go-wrong colors: The first step is to decide whether your skin contains more red (ruddy) or yellow (sallow) tones, says Geller. (If you can't tell, hold a piece of very white paper against your skin. It will help you to see these red or yellow tones.)

Yellow-based shades such as gold beige or honey beige are most flattering to ruddy skin, while rosier shades such as rose beige and ivory beige can perk up a sallow complexion, says Geller. Very fair skin is most flattered by shades that look more ivory than yellow, such as alabaster.

Test makeup on your chest or neck, rather than on your hand. "The skin in these areas is a closer match to skin on your face," says Milek.

Perfect application: Apply an oil-based foundation with a wet cosmetic sponge, says Milek. "It goes on more thinly and evenly that way." Sponge on a bit more foundation on areas of discoloration—for most of us, the cheeks and the sides of the nose.

Don't use too much foundation under your eyes. "A thick layer of foundation in this area will draw attention to crow's-feet and skin that's gotten a little mottled like crepe paper," she says.

Tips and tricks: To get the look of flawless skin without using a ton of foundation, use your fingers to smooth a small amount just over your cheeks or the sides of your nose, suggests Geller. Blend well so that you can't see where the foundation begins and ends.

Concealer: The Great Cover-Up

Remember when concealer had the consistency and color of Spackle? Not anymore. These days, concealers are lighter and creamier, and they come in almost as many shades as foundations do.

Most flattering formulation: Choose a creamy concealer that comes in a pot or with a wand (such as Almay Extra Moisturizing Undereye Cover Cream or Almay Time-Off Age-Smoothing Concealer). They're sheerer and lighter than stick formulations, so they won't look thick or chalky when you wear them. They're also easier to blend than stick concealers and won't drag across the thin, delicate skin under the eyes.

Can't-go-wrong colors: Choose a concealer one shade lighter than your skin tone, says Geller. To find a perfect match, go to a store where samples are available, then dab a bit on your cheek and head outside (or to a window)

with your compact so that you can view the shade in broad daylight. (As awkward as this sounds, you'll only have to do it once.)

Perfect application: Apply concealer *after* foundation. "This way, if your foundation covers the flaw, you can skip it altogether," says Geller.

Here's how to camouflage dark circles, a common problem for women with mature skin, says Geller. Using a small, soft brush or your finger, dot a tiny amount of concealer under each eye, from the inside corner to the middle. (Don't extend it to the outside of the eye because it will eventually seep into crow's-feet.) Then blend the product into your foundation with your finger or a tiny brush until you can't see it anymore. Blot off the excess with a tissue or cotton square.

Tips and tricks: If the skin under your eyes is very dry, pat on a light eye cream before you apply concealer, says Geller. It will make even a sheer concealer sheerer.

Blush: How to Get Glowing Again

As we get older, skin often becomes more sallow. But no one has to know. Properly selected and applied, blusher can help mature skin recapture the rosiness of youth.

Most flattering formulation: Blushers come in cream, powder, and cream-powder formulations. Cream formulations, such as Revlon Colorstay Cheek-color (which comes with a sponge rather than a brush), or cream-powder blushers are most flattering to dry or mature skin. "Powder blushers accentuate lines and wrinkles," says Milek. For sheer, "barely there" color, try a gel, such as Origins Pinch Your Cheeks (available in some department stores).

Can't-go-wrong colors: Warm shades of blush that contain more yellow than red are more forgiving of mature skin. "Virtually any woman looks beautiful in warm shades of peach and pink," Milek says.

If you have gray hair, use shades of pink, rose, plum, or mauve. "They complement gray hair beautifully, no matter what your skin tone," says Geller.

Perfect application: If you need to minimize lines and wrinkles, apply blusher to the apples of your cheeks only, says Geller. (To find this point, smile broadly, then find the swell with your fingers.)

GETTING THE LIPS YOU WANT

As we age, we may lose pigment in our skin and lips. Some women also notice that their upper lips get thinner.

To counteract the effects of time and get fuller-looking lips, choose light- to medium-colored lipstick and a matching lip liner. Keep in mind that lighter colors tend to make lips appear larger and fuller, while darker colors will shrink them. The same goes for lip liner, says Pat Ely, a makeup artist in Walnut Creek, California. "A lot of women like to use a dark liner to outline their lips, thinking it will make them stand out, but darker colors will only make lips look smaller."

Instead, match your liner to your lipstick, adding a spot of glossy color to your bottom lip for a fuller effect. Outline your mouth with lip liner and fill in with a matching lipstick. If you're not happy with the natural shape of your mouth, says Ely, apply the lip liner slightly outside of your natural lip line.

To make your bottom lip look fuller, use a lighter shade of frosted or glossy lip color in the center of your lower lip.

To apply cream blusher, place a dime-size dot on each cheek with a finger or a cosmetic sponge, says Geller. Then blend, wiping off excess color with a piece of tissue or a cotton square. To apply cream-powder blusher, touch the bristles of the brush to the product, tap off the excess color, and apply lightly. Blend until you can't see where the color begins or ends.

Tips and tricks: While powder blushers are beautiful, many contain intense pigment and end up looking too dark, says Milek. To tone down the color of your favorite powder blush, dip your blusher brush into a little loose powder (baby powder is fine), then apply the blusher itself.

Powder: Set It and Forget It

Despite what you may think, using powder will *not* draw attention to your every line and wrinkle, says Milek. "Used correctly, powder sets makeup and gives it a polished look," she says.

Most flattering formulation:
Powders come in two formulations—
pressed or loose—and both can be used
on mature skin, says Milek. Pressed
powder comes in a compact and is applied with a dry sponge. Loose powder
comes in a container and is brushed on
with a large, fluffy brush.

Whichever formulation you choose,
buy a product made specifically for
mature skin: They contain added moisturizers. Two to try are Revlon Age-
Defying Pressed Loose Powder and
Maybelline Moisture Whip Loose
Powder.

Can't-go-wrong colors: Select a
powder three shades lighter than your
foundation, says Milek. If you don't
wear foundation, dust your face with a
sheer, tinted, loose or pressed powder
to hide flaws and give skin a more polished appearance, suggests Geller.

Perfect application: To apply
pressed powder, "tap" the powder into
your makeup using the puff that comes
with the compact, says Milek.

Dust on loose powder with a big,
fluffy makeup brush, whisking off the
excess. Once a week, clean your powder
brush in warm, soapy water. A clean
brush slips across your skin better than
one permeated with facial oil, says Milek.

Before you touch up your makeup,
blend foundation that has seeped into
the lines around your eyes and mouth
with a dry sponge or a piece of tissue,
advises Milek. "If you don't, your
powder will set those creases," she says.

Tips and tricks: For special occasions, dust
a lightly frosted powder over your cheekbones,
suggests Geller. "It will give your skin an
added glow."

REAL-LIFE SCENARIO

She's Never Worn Makeup and Doesn't Know Where to Start

Marti had one of those "peaches 'n' cream" complexions
when she was younger, firm and unblemished, with lively,
impish green eyes and full lips that seemed to curve up at
the edges, as if she were smiling at a secret. Her mother
would never let her wear makeup. Someone so fresh,
healthy, and full of color didn't need it. Only now that she's
in her forties, she does need it. Her eyes, once so bright,
seem washed out. Her complexion has become pale and
dry. Her lips have grown thinner. Her friends have encouraged her to start wearing a little makeup, but when she tried
applying foundation, lipstick, eyeliner, and rouge, they made
her look even older. She's not discouraged yet, but she
doesn't know what to try next. Is there a good place for her
to start?

The truth is, applying makeup is a
skill, and as with any skill, practice makes perfect. Marti will
need to experiment with makeup until she hits upon products that suit her skin and she finds her own unique
makeup style.

Marti will save money and learn more quickly if she ex-
periments with one or two cosmetics at a time. Lipstick
and mascara are makeup basics, so she should focus on
them first.

Finding the "right" lipstick is a matter of trial and error,
even for women who've used cosmetics for years. But in
general, cream lipsticks in soft, warm shades soften the look
of aging skin and play down lines around the mouth.

If Marti has tiny vertical lines around her mouth, using a
colorless (nude) lip pencil will keep her lipstick from
bleeding. Nude shades are virtually invisible, so they're most
forgiving of shaky fingers.

Eye Makeup: Pump Up Your Peeper Power

A soft smudge of liner around your eyes and a
coat or two of mascara can make your eyes ap-

As for mascara, Marti should avoid the "thickening" formulas. Many contain fibers that can make lashes look clumpy and messy. To thicken her lashes, she can dust them with powder first, then apply mascara.

Blush comes next. Because Marti has dry skin, she should opt for a cream blush that closely matches the shade of her lipstick.

Finding the right foundation can be tricky, but once Marti finds it, chances are she'll never have to do it again.

An oil-based foundation makes dry skin look fresher and gives it a dewy appearance. To find the right shade, Marti should match the foundation to the skin on her neck—in natural light, if possible.

Sometimes, makeup-shy women don't like the feel of foundation on their skin. To get the look of flawless skin without feeling as though she's wearing a mask, Marti can apply foundation only to areas of discoloration—on most women, the cheeks, around the nose, under the eyes, and the chin, blending until she can't see where the foundation begins and ends.

Makeup novices often end their foundation at their jawlines. If Marti wants to use foundation all over her face, she'll need to use it on the entire front of her neck, too. Using a makeup sponge moistened with water will help her blend flawlessly and give her foundation a sheer, "barely there" look.

Marti can tackle eye shadow and other eye makeup later on, when she's mastered the basics. It shouldn't be long until she's using makeup with confidence and looking more youthful.

Expert consulted
Paula Mayer
Makeup artist
San Diego

pear bigger and brighter. And if you have droopy lids, a subtle application of the right eye shadow can help bring them out of hiding.

Most flattering formulation: The skin around our eyes becomes thinner and drier with age. Cream-based eye shadows and pencils will nourish this delicate skin while they camouflage crinkles.

Eye shadow. Eye shadows come in two basic formulations. Cream shadows (such as Revlon Age-Defying Eye Color) are usually applied with a wand. Powder shadows come in a cake and are applied with a sponge-tip applicator or a brush. If your skin is very dry, opt for cream-based shadows, says Geller. "They're easy to apply and long wearing," she adds. And like cream blushers, creamy shadows soften the appearance of wrinkles.

Also, select a shadow with a bit of shimmer to it—in makeup artist jargon, a "low-pearl" shadow. Yes, you heard right. "Most women think that frosted shadows will accentuate aging eyes," says Geller. "In fact, a softly shimmering shadow can soften them." Avoid Las Vegas–showgirl frosts, however. Very sparkly, glittery shadows spotlight every droop and wrinkle.

Eyeliner. Opt for pencil liners, recommends Geller. Wax-based eye pencils are fine, but the softer ones may smudge, and the extra-hard ones will drag across delicate undereye skin. So she recommends using powder eyeliner pencils (such as Elizabeth Arden Smoky Eyes Powder Pencil or Revlon Softsmoke Powderliner). "They make the eyes look smoky and soft, and they're easy to apply," she says.

What *not* to use: liquid liners. "If you have lines on your face, you don't need to paint on more," says Milek.

Mascara. Choose a fiber-free mascara. Most mascara is fiber-free, but if not, the packaging will be labeled "with fibers," Geller says. Mascaras that contain fibers tend to cake, clump, and look goopy, which draws attention to aging eyes.

Can't-go-wrong colors: Afraid you'll use the wrong shade of shadow or pencil and end up looking like, well, your eccentric Aunt Matilda? You won't if you use muted hues that flatter your hair color and skin tone.

Eye shadow. Those of us with dark hair and medium to dark skin can wear virtually any shade of shadow. "Brunettes look particularly good in bronze or champagne, which is a very pale pink," says Geller. Blondes with ruddy skin look best in shades of taupe, beige, and charcoal brown, while blondes with more yellow in their skin are flattered by shades of violet, slate, and gray-brown. If you have gray hair, you'll always look great in shades of taupe and soft gray, she says.

Eyeliner. Darker shades of navy and hunter green flatter any skin tone and make the whites of the eyes appear brighter, says Geller. For a more subtle effect, use shades of brown or khaki (a soft greenish brown). If you're using black liner, toss it immediately: "Black is much too harsh for mature skin," she says.

Mascara. Black for brunettes, brown for blondes and redheads, says Geller. To give your eyes an extra sparkle, try navy mascara. "It adds just a hint of color and will make your eyes appear brighter," she says.

Perfect application: Applying shadow, liner, and mascara to your best advantage can be tricky, but using the tips below will make the job much easier.

Eye shadow. To apply a cream-based shadow, smudge it on with a clean pinky finger, says Milek. "It's easier to control your finger than an applicator, and the color will be softer and more subtle," she says.

Stroke on powder shadow with a small eye brush. "A brush distributes the color more finely and evenly than a sponge applicator can," says Geller. Brush a V-shaped arc of shadow from the outer corner of your eye, extending one side of the V so that the shadow covers any drooping area over the lid and brushing the other side into your lashes.

Eyeliner. If you have shaky fingers, apply eye makeup sitting at a table, using a mirror placed at eye level, suggests Geller. Rest the elbow of the hand holding the eye pencil on the table. Then anchor your elbow with your other hand.

Mascara. For clump-free lashes, wipe off the wand before applying mascara, says Milek. To thicken skimpy lashes, dust them with powder before you apply the first coat.

Tips and tricks: Curling your lashes will make them appear thicker and your eyes bigger and brighter, says Milek.

Dig out your metal eyelash curler—the one you swore you'd never use again—and hold it under your blow-dryer for 5 to 10 seconds. The heat will help your lashes hold their curl, says Geller. (Use common sense, please: Test the metal against your hand before touching it to your eye area.)

Lipstick: The Bare Essential

"Every woman should wear lipstick, regardless of her age," says Geller. "But if you have mature skin, the right lipstick can brighten up your entire face, making your skin appear more youthful."

Most flattering formulation: Lips get drier with age. To keep them moist and supple, choose cream lipsticks, which contain added moisturizers (such as Revlon Moon Drops Moisture Creme and Lancôme Hydra-Riche Hydrating Lip Colour), advises Geller. As a bonus, cream formulations soften the appearance of mature skin and draw attention away from lines and wrinkles, she says.

If you prefer a more natural look, try lip gloss. "It provides just a hint of color and a faint shimmer," says Milek.

Can't-go-wrong colors: If you're a fair-skinned blonde, opt for soft shades of mauve (warm pink), says Paula Mayer, a makeup artist in San Diego. Blondes with darker skin look great in warm browns, such as sand, or orange-based reds. Olive-skinned brunettes look best in shades of peach, orange-red, wine, and burgundy. Fair-skinned brunettes should favor bright fuchsias or softer shades of pink. Redheads with freckles look best in cinnamon and terra cotta colors.

Shades of mauve, apricot, and copper will "cool down" ruddy skin or deemphasize broken capillaries, adds Milek.

All of us can wear what's called a true red, which contains an equal amount of yellow and

---

HOW TO BE A SMASH AT YOUR CLASS REUNION

Class reunions are a time for fond memories, greeting long-lost friends . . . and worrying about how you're going to look to these people, now that you're 20 or 25 years older. How to look your best? These tips will help you stand out from the crowd around the punch bowl.

Flash a smile in drop-dead red. A woman in red lipstick demands attention, says Laura Geller, makeup artist and owner of Laura Geller Make-Up Studios in New York City. And chances are, it will complement whatever you plan to wear. Red matches especially well with neutral colors such as black, brown, navy, gray, and, well, red. Forget the red lips, though, if you plan to wear an unusual color, such as purple or orange.

Shape up those brows. Now is a perfect opportunity to have your eyebrows professionally waxed and shaped, says Geller, especially if they're on the bushy side. "Neat, well-groomed eyebrows emphasize your eyes," she says. Depending on where you live, this little luxury could cost you less than $15.

Be perfectly polished. As long as you're getting your brows done, treat yourself to a professional manicure, too, says Judith Ann Graham, vice president of the Association of Image Consultants International in Washington, D.C. "You'll be holding and hugging people, and your hands will be on display."

Sport a jacket. Consider wearing a pantsuit with a jacket. "Wearing a jacket makes a statement: 'I'm powerful, in control,'" says Graham. That's not to say you should wear your interview suit. "An elegant, feminine pantsuit in a color you love can make you look powerful, yet still approachable," she says.

blue. "True red lipstick looks particularly striking on women with gray hair," says Milek. Another foolproof color, according to Milek: Natural Mist Cream, made by Sally Hansen. "It's not brown, it's not peach, it's not pink, but a combination of the three. And it works on every woman," she says.

Whatever color you choose, stick to soft shades. "Lips get thinner with age," says Geller. "Very dark colors make them look even thinner."

Perfect application: Most of us slick on lipstick straight from the tube. Perfectly fine, says Geller. But if your lip color seeps into tiny creases above your lips, enlist the aid of a lip pencil, she advises. "The wax in the pencil acts as a barrier, keeping lipstick from feathering or bleeding," she says. For a soft, natural look, use a nude lip liner.

Tips and tricks: To plump up thin lips, choose a lip color with just a hint of frost. "Soft frosts reflect light, which makes lips appear fuller," says Geller.

To keep lipstick off your teeth, do what models do: After you apply lipstick, put your index finger in your mouth. Then draw it out slowly, with your mouth closed. "Whatever ends up on your finger would have ended up on your teeth," says Geller. Or you could just swab a little petroleum jelly onto your front upper teeth to keep the lipstick off, she adds.

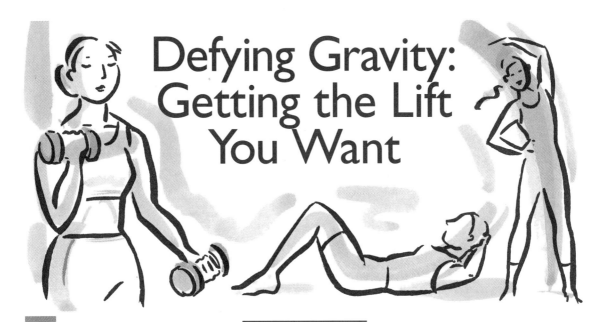

Defying Gravity: Getting the Lift You Want

The average newborn in the United States weighs 7 pounds. The average grocery bag weighs even more. And the average piece of furniture . . . well, women know a lot about heavy lifting.

And since we're doing so much of it anyway, we may as well turn all that lifting to our advantage. After all, if we do it in a regular, organized way, it can make us look younger, feel stronger, and live longer. We don't necessarily want to use the baby, a sack of cantaloupes, or the sofa, of course. Dumbbells are more like what the doctor ordered—and not the kind of dumbbell that gets all your toppings wrong when you order pizza over the telephone, but rather the kind that bodybuilders use.

Pump Iron to Stop the Clock

Did the word *bodybuilder* make you cringe? Don't worry. You won't bulk up like a female Arnold Schwarzenegger. Instead, you'll slow the sagging and bulging that begins as gravity starts to get the better of us in our midthirties. That's when many of us start to lose one-fourth to one-third of a pound of muscle every year and replace it with fat because of slowing metabolism and a less active lifestyle.

The problem is that fat takes up more space than muscle, so even if you don't gain a pound, your clothes will gradually feel tighter as you grow older. It doesn't look good, and it doesn't feel good.

So if the problem is to keep fat off, why don't we just diet?

It's true that as we get older, we can ward off wiggly arms and thighs by controlling our weight. But eventually, even thin women will see signs of sagging. That's where strength training comes in. "I think if there's one thing that really is the elixir of youth for women as they age, it's strength training," says Joan Price, a certified fitness instructor, speaker, and writer from Sebastopol, California, and author of *Joan Price Says, Yes, You Can Get in Shape!*

Shed Excuses, Shed Years

But I'm too old to start lifting weights. Is that what you're thinking? Think again.

"We have women in their nineties who are strength-training and doing really well," says Miriam E. Nelson, Ph.D., director of the Center for Physical Fitness at Tufts University School of Nutrition Science and Policy in Boston and author of *Strong Women Stay Slim* and *Strong Women Stay Young.* "Certainly, we love for women to start at a younger age, but if you're already 75 or 92, then that's the right age to start."

Okay, maybe I'm not too old, but I'm barely able to take the time to eat, let alone spend a few hours in a leotard lifting weights at a gym. This is an excellent excuse. You're to be commended. Unfortunately, it won't work. Just ditch the leotard and plan to stay home.

All it takes to tone your trouble zones are two or three at-home sessions a week. You can even break up the sessions into smaller workouts. Best of all, you will see dramatic changes in your body in about a month, and most women get a big energy boost right away, says Dr. Nelson.

More Than Skin Deep

The benefits to resistance training go way beyond reshaping your body.

A study done by Dr. Nelson and her colleagues at the Jean Mayer USDA Human Nutrition Research Center on Aging at Tufts University found that 20 women who began a strength-training program sometime after menopause completely transformed their bodies—inside and out. After a year of doing a five-exercise workout twice a week, the women were in the same physical condition as women 15 to 20 years younger, says Dr. Nelson. Here are some of the anti-aging benefits these women gained from strength training.

REAL-LIFE SCENARIO

Is She Destined to Look Like Her Mom?

Every time Nancy, 44, looks at her mom, she gets a sinking feeling in the pit of her stomach. What she sees is a woman, only in her sixties, who is hunched over, shuffling in her step, overweight, and covered with age spots. Her mother's face seems leathery and more wrinkled than it ought to be, covered with fine lines, especially around the lips. What unsettles Nancy most is looking through old family albums. Her mother had been such a beauty. There's one picture, in particular, of her lounging on a veranda in a hotel in sunny Puerto Rico, a martini in one hand and a cigarette in the other, and the most dazzling smile on her face. She was breathtaking, sophisticated. But that person seemed to have disappeared entirely over the years, and in her place is a woman whom Nancy still very much loves ... but doesn't want to become. She's desperate to find some way to avoid her mother's fate.

Nancy is not on a predestined path to premature aging. Although genetics *do* play a role in how we look as we age, the health and lifestyle habits we follow when we're younger can determine much of how we look when we're older.

The photo of Nancy's mother reveals several habits that may have added years to her appearance.

For starters, smoking can cause premature and pronounced wrinkling—especially around the lips—because it robs the skin of two things it needs to be healthy: oxygen and vitamin C. Not to mention that smoking increases your risk for more serious conditions, such as heart disease and cancer. Her mother's smoking habit also may have contributed to her hunched-over posture, which is a sign of osteoporosis. That's a condition that turns your bones so brittle that they easily break. Smoking weakens your skeleton in two ways: It interferes with bone formation and promotes bone loss. Because osteoporosis is often genetic, Nancy may be at increased risk. But she can reduce her risk by not smoking and by getting 1,000 milligrams of calcium a day through diet and supplements.

The martini in her mother's hand may seem innocent enough, but regular alcohol intake can weaken bones and contribute to wrinkling as well. And alcoholic beverages are loaded with "empty" calories, meaning they provide no nutrition, which may have led to another one of her mother's problems—weight gain. To protect her bones and maintain her weight, Nancy should stick to drinking no more than one alcoholic drink a day.

From the photo, it appears her mother was also a sun worshiper. Sun damage is the number one cause of wrinkles and leathery skin—as well as those age spots. Unprotected exposure to the sun can also lead to skin cancer. For the health of her skin, Nancy should avoid sunbathing and should wear sunscreen with a sun protection factor (SPF) of at least 15 whenever she goes outdoors.

Another important stay-young strategy is regular exercise. Aerobic exercise combined with strength training can help Nancy maintain her weight, prevent osteoporosis, and improve her posture and balance—so instead of shuffling, she'll be *springing* in her step when she hits 60.

Expert consulted
Clarita E. Herrera, M.D.
Clinical instructor of primary care
New York Medical College
Valhalla

Thinner physique. The women in the study were told to stick with their normal diet so that they wouldn't gain or lose weight during the 1-year period. The women doing the strength training may not have dropped pounds, but they lost fat and gained muscle. They looked much leaner, and some even dropped as many as two dress sizes.

Higher metabolism. Although your metabolism tends to slow down as you get older, making it more difficult to maintain your weight, there are ways to speed it up again. Increasing the amount of muscle you have is one. That's because muscle tissue burns more calories than fat. One woman in the study gave her metabolism a major boost: She lost 29 pounds of fat and, as a result, now burns 160 extra calories a day.

Increased strength. Dr. Nelson's study showed that within 2 months, women typically double the amount of weight they can lift. That's good news for a lot of people. According to one study of 10,000 women ages 40 to 55, more than one-fourth struggle with everyday tasks such as carrying groceries or walking up a flight of stairs.

More energy. As the women in Dr. Nelson's study became stronger, they felt more energized and began doing things that they hadn't done in years—or had never done at all. They went canoeing, river rafting, dancing, bicycle riding, and skating. By the end of the study, the women in the strength-training group were 27 percent more active than a year before, while the group that hadn't done strength training had become 25 percent *less* active in that year.

Improved mood. Lifting weights can lift your spirits. In another study conducted at the same USDA laboratory, strength training was found to be comparable to antidepressant drugs at fighting depression, which affects far more women than men.

Added bone. After menopause, women typically lose 1 percent of their bone mass each year. Over time, eight million women develop osteoporosis, a condition in which bones become so brittle that they easily break. The strength-training group in Dr. Nelson's study *gained* 1 percent of bone density, while those who didn't strength-train *lost* about 2 percent.

Better balance. Our balance deteriorates as we age, making us more likely to suffer a bad fall. The women in the study who didn't do strength training experienced an 8½ percent decline in balance, while those who lifted weights improved their balance by 14 percent.

Gearing Up: What You Need to Get Started

For hundreds of dollars less than a one-year gym membership, you can buy everything you need to start our body-shaping program now. And just imagine what you'll save on leotards. Here's how to equip yourself.

Pick up some dumbbells. Also called free weights, they are available in 1-pound increments from 1 to 20 pounds. Beginners may want to start out with lighter weights. Pairs of 3-, 5-, 8-, and 10-pound dumbbells should do the job and will run anywhere from around $25 to $55 for all four pairs. They even come in pretty pastel colors.

SHAPE UP WITH THE STARS

How do Hollywood celebs keep their sleek physiques? With a hot strengthening and stretching program called the Pilates Method of Body Conditioning.

This method, developed over 70 years ago by German gymnast, boxer, and circus performer Joseph Pilates, caught on in the 1950s among top dancers who wanted to stay in shape and prevent injury. Unlike most exercise programs, Pilates simultaneously works on strength, flexibility, and balance. Now it's toning up stunning stars like Madonna, Sharon Stone, Jane Seymour, Vanessa Williams, Uma Thurman, Julia Roberts, and Jodie Foster. What's more, because of its effect on conditioning, suppleness, and balance, it may be one secret to staying young.

The Pilates Method (pronounced "puh-LAH-teez") promises to make you look taller and leaner and to build strength and flexibility—without developing bodybuilder-size muscles. It will leave you with a slimmer shape, improve your posture and balance, and give better overall function to your body. And best of all, you'll start to see results in a matter of weeks. The method's inventor offers this guarantee: "You will feel better in 10 sessions, look better in 20 sessions, and have a completely new body in 30 sessions."

Here's how it works. Each session lasts 45 minutes to an hour and takes you through a series of precise, controlled movements that require concentration and controlled breathing. The main focus of the Pilates Method is to

---

Purchase some padding. A foam mat can turn any floor into a home gym. Mats are great for floor stretches, pushups, and crunches, and they cost around $10.

Have a seat. You will need a sturdy chair without arms for at least one exercise we describe later. A few others—such as the biceps curl and the overhead press—can be done either standing or seated. A chair from your dining room set may fill the bill.

strengthen the "powerhouse" of your anatomy—the abdomen, lower back, and buttocks—to enable the rest of your body to move more freely. You use continuous, flowing movements and low repetitions to tone without bulking. There are 19 apparatuses with unusual names like Pedipull, Reformer, and Cadillac, which help strengthen your muscles through a full range of motion. Or you can do your entire workout on a mat. Ideally, you should do two to three sessions per week.

The method incorporates 500 exercises, but you'll probably only do 30 to 40 per session and may only learn a total of 50 to 60. That's because certified Pilates trainers design a workout to meet your personal fitness goals.

"This is probably the most widely adaptable exercise system that's available today," says Sean P. Gallagher, a physical therapist and national director of the Pilates Studio in New York City. "You can use this system whether you're completely out of shape or you're a superstar athlete. I've worked with amputees, people with head injuries, young people, and even people in their eighties."

Women who've tried Pilates rave about the results. After just 40 sessions, 49-year-old Patricia Scanlon of Philadelphia feels more than a decade younger. "My waist is smaller, my stomach is tighter, my posture is better, and I'm stronger and more energetic," she says. "The strengthening you do with Pilates is so deep. I'm getting down into muscles I never felt before. It's sort of like a massage from the inside out."

Dress the part. As promised, no leotard. But you will need a pair of athletic shoes. "A good pair of athletic shoes offers both stability when you're doing the exercises and some protection, just in case you drop a free weight," says Price. You should also wear comfortable clothes made of a breathable fabric like a cotton/synthetic blend.

"Avoid wearing anything that could impair your range of motion or anything so baggy that a weight could become lodged in your clothing," says John Duncan, Ph.D., an exercise physiologist at Texas Woman's University Center for Research on Women's Health in Denton.

Strength Training 101

Like any sport or activity, strength training has tricks to learn and techniques to master. Strength training can involve using weights or your own body weight to challenge and build muscle. Here's a quick lesson to help you get the most from your workout.

Know the lingo. The words *rep* and *set* are the jargon of gym junkies. We will decode them for you. One rep, or repetition, describes one complete exercise. So one pushup, for example, would be one rep. A set is just that—a set of repetitions. Dr. Nelson recommends doing two sets of 8 to 12 repetitions for each exercise. Start with 8 repetitions in each set. When you can easily do 12, you can add a little more weight.

Work out between meals. Right after eating a Thanksgiving feast is not the best time to pick up a pair of dumbbells. "If your stomach is really full, you're going to feel uncomfortable," Dr. Nelson says. It is also unwise to work out when you haven't eaten for several hours. "If you're starving, you may get light-headed," she says. To be at your best, try to work out midway between meals or have a light meal or snack an hour or so beforehand.

Warm up. We're not talking about drinking hot cocoa by a toasty fire. We mean warming up your muscles for 5 to 10 minutes so that you don't go directly from sitting in front of the TV to lifting 12-pound weights over your head. Muscles much prefer being eased into exercise. To warm up, you can take a brisk walk, do jumping jacks, march or jog in place, or do toning exercises for 5 to 10 reps without weights. If you do an aerobic workout in addition to resistance training, says Dr. Nelson, you can do the aerobics first, in place of a warmup.

Pick the right weight. If you lift weights that are too heavy, you could hurt yourself. On the other hand, lifting weights that are too light won't do much to firm your flab. Here's a good rule of thumb: If you can't lift the weight in good form 8 times, then it's too heavy, Dr. Nelson says. But if you can easily lift the weight more than 12 times, it's too light.

Lift with a friend. Beginners may want to find a weight buddy. That person serves three purposes. First, she can lend a hand if you tire and struggle through that last repetition, Dr. Duncan says. Second, she can watch to make sure that you are using good form. And third, she can offer the encouragement that first-time lifters often need.

Don't wait to exhale. Strange as it may sound, many weight lifters literally hold their breath, which can cause their blood pressures to spike. The proper way to breathe, says Dr. Nelson, is to exhale on the exertion—when you lift the weight or do the crunch—and inhale as you lower the weight or return to the starting position.

PERK UP YOUR POSTURE

Let's play detective. We walk along a dimly lit street and see two feminine figures looming in the shadows. Without seeing their faces, it's clear that one woman is far older than the other. What gives away her age? Posture. One woman stands straight as a pencil and the other bends over like a banana.

The good news is that even banana-shaped women can take steps to straighten up—and there are plenty of reasons to undo the hunch. For starters, correct posture prevents muscle and bone pain and allows us to breathe properly. Standing up straight can make us look taller, thinner, younger, and more confident. And good posture helps our clothing to fit its best. That's because clothes are cut for people with "normal" posture, says Margit L. Bleecker, M.D., Ph.D., director of the Center for Occupational and Environmental Neurology in Baltimore.

But we don't have to have the posture of a ballerina to reap the benefits. "There is no such thing as perfect posture," Dr. Bleecker says. "There's a spectrum of what is acceptable posture." A good rule is to keep your ears, shoulders, hips, knees, and ankles in a straight line as much as possible. Doing so can actually *prevent* the unsightly slump. That's because women who have good posture before they hit menopause—when their bones start to demineralize—are less likely to end up hunched over, she says.

But if your posture needs perking up, one easy way to do that is to adjust your work habits. If you do a lot of computer work, for example, take short breaks. "Working at a keyboard promotes poor posture, so it's important to stand up whenever possible and move around," Dr. Bleecker says.

If you have a job that requires you to stand most of the day, such as working a cash register, try putting one foot up on a box or telephone book. "When standing for a long time, the lower back tends to arch and the hips lean forward," Dr. Bleecker explains. "Elevating one foot can prevent this."

Correcting poor posture may also mean doing a balancing act. "Most posture problems are caused by an imbalance of muscles," Dr. Bleecker says. Women who tend to bend slightly forward as they stand usually have tight, shortened muscles in the front of their bodies and weak, elongated muscles in the back. Stretching the tight muscles and strengthening the weak ones with the proper exercises can help stop the slump.

Perhaps most important, we should pay attention to how we're sitting, standing, and walking and make any necessary adjustments to correct our posture. After a while, it will become automatic. When sitting at your computer, keep your back in contact with the chair and your feet flat on the floor. Your thighs should be parallel with the floor, and your shoulders should stay relaxed, with your elbows at a right angle to your body.

Tame the tension. "When we contract one muscle, we have a tendency to tense the others as well. But during strength training, only the muscles you're working should contract," writes Dr. Nelson in her book *Strong Women Stay Young*. Some common trouble spots to check: Make sure that you're not clenching your teeth, furrowing your brow, or tensing your shoulders up around your ears.

Take it slow. Fast, herky-jerky movements can cause injury. They can also cause you to use momentum, rather than muscle, to lift weight. Slow, controlled movements, on the other hand, are safer and take more effort—so you get more benefit, Price says. Each repetition should take about 6 seconds: 2 seconds to lift the weight, a 2-second pause, and then another 2 seconds to lower the weight.

Perfect your form. Good form—doing an exercise in exactly the right way—helps you get the most benefit from lifting and prevents injury, says Price. An easy way to watch your lifting form is to position yourself in front of a full-length mirror. Make sure that your wrists are straight, not bent backward or forward. And be sure that you are doing the exercise precisely as it is shown.

Pay attention to posture. Whether you're sitting or standing when you lift dumbbells, keep your back, neck, and head straight to prevent muscle strain and injury. And good posture doesn't mean standing stiff. Stand tall but relaxed. If you're

WOMAN TO WOMAN

She Looks and Feels Far Younger Than Her Years

Filomena Warihay, president of an international consulting firm in Downingtown, Pennsylvania, still slips into her size 4 bikini at age 61. But she hasn't always been so fit and trim. Her body was slowly giving in to time and gravity, when a chance invitation from her daughter introduced her to a whole new way of life. From that day on, her body seemed to grow younger. Here's her story.

I haven't always had the body I have today. I really struggled to fit in workouts when I had four small children to take care of. I would sit them in a wagon and pull them up and down the street to get in a walk. I parked my car a mile from work and walked the rest of the way.

Then, when I was 40, one of my daughters was awarded a full athletic scholarship to college. When she received her summer training schedule, she realized that she'd have to go to the gym 3 days a week. She begged me to go with her. I did, but my primary motivation was to help her get her college education paid for.

After we'd gone to the gym for a while, my daughter said, "Mom, I bet you could run a mile." Well, I tried, and I couldn't. We went over to the track, and it was pitiful. But we stayed with it, and by the middle of the summer, I ran in a local 5-K race. To my surprise, I came in second or third in my age category. I've won a medal in that race every year since.

Now I'm even more disciplined about exercising. I work out 6 days a week, either running 6 miles outdoors, chugging away on my stairclimber, or going to the gym. I lift weights and do 400 crunches every other day and stretch daily for about 15 minutes. I actually feel better now than when I was 30. And I'm within 5 pounds of what I weighed when I graduated from high school.

Most people think I'm in my forties, and I'm not ashamed to tell them the truth. Nor am I embarrassed to wear any of my six or so bikinis. Still, every year I say to my husband, "Maybe this is the last year I'll be able to wear a bikini." And he always says, "I'll tell you when."

seated to do the exercise, sit up straight with your feet flat on the floor, recommends Dr. Nelson.

Be kind to your joints. Avoid locking your elbows or knees when lifting weights. "Anytime you lock a joint, the joint bears the stress of the weight, not the muscle," Price says. "To prevent joint pain, end the move just short of locking your knees or elbows."

Break between sets. Take a 1- to 2-minute break after completing each set to give your muscles a chance to recuperate and prepare for the next set. To save time, Dr. Nelson points out, you can do an exercise that works another muscle group. Try alternating between leg and arm exercises, for example.

Finish with flexibility. The ideal time to stretch is after your workout, when your muscles are warmed up. Lifting weights actually contracts and shortens your muscles, making them less flexible. But stretching after lifting restores muscle length and keeps them supple, which prevents injury in the long run. "When you're inflexible, you're much more prone to injury," Dr. Nelson says, "because instead of your muscles being elastic and allowing some give, they're quite tight."

Take a day off. Your muscles need at least a day to rest in between resistance-training sessions. It's actually during that time that your muscles get stronger, Dr. Nelson says. That's because lifting weights causes tiny tears in the muscle tissue. As your muscles repair that damage, they become stronger, she explains.

Work through soreness. You're probably going to feel a little sore for the first few weeks after starting a new body-toning program. Only when the soreness subsides should you increase the amount of weight you're lifting, and then add no more than a pound per session. If the soreness is significant, so that even everyday movement is painful, you may need to decrease the weight, says Dr. Nelson.

Mix up your routine. After lifting weights consistently for a few weeks or months, you may hit a plateau. That's when you find that you can't seem to progress to the next level with heavier weights. This is a sign that your muscles have become used to your workout and need a new challenge to grow further. "When you hit a plateau, try changing something in your routine," Price suggests.

Alter the exercise slightly, try a completely different exercise to work the same muscle, or lift and lower the weight even more slowly. For example, take 4 seconds to lift the weight, a 2-second pause, and then 4 seconds to lower it.

Pay attention to pain. Pain may be a sign that a muscle, tendon, or joint has been overworked or strained. "If something doesn't feel right, don't keep training it," Dr. Nelson says. Rest a few days before trying your routine again.

STOP THE SAG

Everything that is tight and firm in our youth starts to sag as we edge over 40. Our bellies. Our butts. Our breasts. Even our skin. Exercise can no doubt help tighten our tummies, derrieres, and chests. But is there a way to tone up sagging skin?

In a word—yes.

Our skin sags as we age for two reasons, says Toby Shawe, M.D., assistant professor of dermatology at the Medical College of Pennsylvania–Hahnemann University Hospitals in Philadelphia. First, the skin's elasticity naturally declines over the years. Second, we tend to gain weight around midlife, which stretches out the skin. If you lose those extra pounds, the decreased elasticity doesn't allow the skin to bounce back as well as it once did. As a result, it will look as though it's sagging—especially in the areas around the belly and butt and under the chin and arms.

To stop the sag before it starts, your best bet is to lose weight very slowly. "Try losing only a pound or two a month," Dr. Shawe says. And while you're losing weight, you can further prevent the sag by toning the underlying muscles with light weight lifting.

Toning those muscles also helps reduce any sagging you may already have. "When the muscle becomes larger, it takes up more space, so the skin won't appear to sag as much," Dr Shawe explains.

And of course, cosmetic surgery to remove the extra skin can help, too. "A combination of surgery and weight lifting often brings women the best results," Dr. Shawe adds.

Give Yourself a Full-Body Face-Lift

With the help of Price and Dr. Nelson, we've put together a total-body workout to firm up all the female trouble spots—the legs, rear end, chest, back, abdomen, shoulders, and arms—so you'll get the best results without putting in hours of effort.

Squat

BODY ZONES TONED: buttocks (gluteus maximus) and thighs (quadriceps and hamstrings)

MASTER THE MOVE: (1) Stand with your feet slightly more than shoulder-width apart. Your toes should point forward or slightly out. Holding the dumbbells, keep your arms straight down at your sides. (2) Keep your back straight, your heels on the floor, and your eyes focused straight ahead. In a slow, controlled movement, lower your body as if you were sitting down in a chair. Sit back over your heels rather than squatting straight down. Your knees should be directly above (never beyond) your toes. Hold for a second and return to the starting position by pushing up from your heels and straightening out your legs. Squeeze your buttock muscles, then repeat.

PLAY IT SAFE: If this is your first time doing resistance training, do this movement without weights for a few sessions. If you feel any stress to the knees, make sure you're sitting back over your heels and not allowing your knees to go beyond your toes. Women who have knee problems should check with their doctors before doing this exercise.

Lunge

BODY ZONES TONED: buttocks (gluteus maximus), thighs (quadriceps and hamstrings), front of hips (hip flexors), and calves (gastrocnemius)

MASTER THE MOVE: (1) Stand with your feet hip-width apart and your arms straight down, holding the dumbbells at your sides. (2) Take a large step forward with your left foot, keeping your back and torso upright and bending both knees. Your left knee should be bent at a 90-degree angle and should not be beyond your toes. Your right knee should be bent a little wider than 90 degrees, and your heel should lift off the floor. Hold for a second and return to the starting position by bringing your back leg forward. Repeat on the opposite side.

PLAY IT SAFE: If you're a beginner, use weights only after you have mastered the move without them. If you have knee problems, check with your doctor before doing this exercise.

Overhead Press

BODY ZONES TONED: shoulders (deltoids), back of upper arms (triceps), and lower neck and upper middle back (trapezius)

MASTER THE MOVE: (1) Start with your feet shoulder-width apart. Hold the dumbbells with your elbows bent and your palms facing front. The inner ends of the dumbbells should touch your shoulders. (2) Push the dumbbells straight up and extend your arms overhead just short of locking your elbows. Slowly lower the dumbbells back to the starting position and repeat.

MIX IT UP: Try changing the move slightly by starting with your palms and forearms facing in toward your chest rather than facing front. As you raise the dumbbells, rotate your forearms and palms so they face front when your arms are extended. Rotate and lower your arms back to the starting position.

Dumbbell Bench Press

BODY ZONES TONED: chest (pectoralis major), front of shoulders (anterior deltoids), and back of upper arms (triceps)

MASTER THE MOVE: (1) Lie back on a bench with your feet flat on the floor. If you find yourself arching your back to reach the floor, put your feet flat on the end of the bench with your knees bent. Keep your buttocks, upper and lower back, and head in line and in contact with the bench during the exercise. Extend your arms above your head with the weights directly above your shoulders and your elbows just short of locking. The inner ends of the dumbbells should touch each other. (2) Slowly lower the dumbbells by bending your elbows and bringing your arms down to your sides. At the end of the move, the weights should be about chest-high and close to your body. Return to the starting position by pushing the dumbbells upward and together. Repeat.

MIX IT UP: If you don't have a workout bench, try lying on a step bench designed for step aerobics.

Pushup

BODY ZONES TONED: chest (pectoralis major), arms (biceps and triceps), and shoulders (deltoids)

MASTER THE MOVE: (1) Lie facedown on an exercise mat with your palms flat on the floor just outside your shoulders. Your fingers should point forward and your elbows should point upward. Bend your legs at the knees so that your feet and lower legs are raised in the air to form a 90-degree angle with your upper legs. (2) Push your torso up. Rest your body weight on the padded part of your lower thigh, slightly above the kneecap. Your thighs, buttocks, back, neck, and head should be in a straight line, and your abdominal muscles should be tight. Make sure that your shoulders are directly above your hands and that your elbows aren't locked. Hold for a second, then lower your torso back to the floor. Repeat.

MIX IT UP: To make this move more difficult, do a full pushup with your legs straight. Only your toes and hands should remain on the floor. Your legs, back, neck, and head should form a straight line.

PLAY IT SAFE: Do not do this exercise if you have carpal tunnel syndrome or if you feel any wrist pain in the pushup position.

Abdominal Crunch

BODY ZONE TONED: abdominals (rectus abdominis)

MASTER THE MOVE: (1) Lie on your back on the exercise mat with your legs bent, keeping your feet flat and your lower back relaxed against the floor. Place your fingers behind your head for support with your elbows pointing out to the sides. Be careful not to pull your head forward with your hands. (2) Use your abdominal muscles to slowly lift your chest and shoulders, making sure not to arch your lower back. Hold for a count of five and slowly return to the starting position. Don't rest between repetitions.

MIX IT UP: For a more advanced workout, lift your lower body toward your chest as you do the crunch. Your legs should be bent slightly at the knees, and your feet should be crossed at the ankles. Raise your torso and lower body at the same time as if you were trying to touch your knees to your shoulders.

PLAY IT SAFE: If you have lower-back pain, try the crunch with your feet and lower legs resting on a chair. Bend your legs at a 90-degree angle, and keep your lower back against the floor when you do the move.

Triceps Extension

BODY ZONES TONED: back of upper arms (triceps)

MASTER THE MOVE: (1) Sit toward the front of a sturdy chair with your back straight and your feet flat on the floor. Bring the arm holding the dumbbell straight up over your head. Bend your arm at the elbow and slowly lower the weight back to your shoulder as far as is comfortable. Keep your elbow close to your ear and pointed toward the ceiling. Support your lifting arm near the elbow with your free hand. (2) Keeping your upper arm still, raise your lower arm over your head just short of locking your elbow. Lower the weight back to the starting position and repeat. Switch arms for the next set.

Biceps Curl

BODY ZONES TONED: front of upper arms (biceps)

MASTER THE MOVE: (1) Stand with your feet about shoulder-width apart and with your arms straight down at your sides, holding the dumbbells so that your palms are facing your thighs. (2) Lift the weights in one smooth motion by bending your elbows, rotating your forearms so that your palms face up, and raising the dumbbells to shoulder height. Keep your wrists and back straight. Slowly lower the weights back to the starting position and repeat.

MIX IT UP: To make this move more difficult, try what is called a concentration curl. Sit on the end of a bench or chair with your feet flat on the ground and your legs bent at a 90-degree angle. Your feet should be slightly more than shoulder-width apart. Hold a dumbbell in one hand. Lean your torso forward a bit and rest the elbow and upper arm you are working against your inner thigh. Keep your free hand on your other knee for support. Slowly lift the dumbbell to your shoulder, keeping your elbow and upper arm firm against your thigh.

Stretch Your Limits

Follow your workout with these stretches to increase your flexibility and lower your risk of injury, says Dr. Nelson.

Lying Quadriceps Stretch

BODY ZONES STRETCHED: front of thighs (quadriceps) and front of hips (hip flexors)

MASTER THE MOVE: Lie on your side with your legs straight and together, one on top of the other. Support your head with the hand closest to the floor by resting your upper arm on the floor and bending it at the elbow. Bend your lower leg slightly if you need to for balance.

Bend the knee of the top leg so that your foot comes back toward your buttocks. Grasp your foot with your free hand and pull the heel in toward your buttocks until you feel a comfortable stretch in the front of your thigh. Hold it there for 20 to 30 seconds, then slowly release. Roll onto your other side and stretch the opposite leg.

Standing Hamstring Stretch

BODY ZONES STRETCHED: back of thighs (hamstrings), inner thighs (adductors), and buttocks (gluteus maximus)

MASTER THE MOVE: Stand with your feet together and take a very large step forward with your right leg. Keep your right foot pointing straight ahead and turn your back leg slightly so that your left foot points a bit to the left.

Bend the knee of your back leg, place your hands on the upper thigh of your front leg, and slowly lean forward with your torso as far as you comfortably can. Keep your back, neck, and head in a straight line. Bend your back leg further while pushing your hips and buttocks down and back. Lift the front of your right foot off the floor, while maintaining pressure on your front heel. You should feel a comfortable stretch in your back and in the inner thigh of your outstretched leg. Hold for 20 to 30 seconds, then stretch the other thigh.

Shoulder Stretch

BODY ZONES STRETCHED: shoulders (deltoids) and arms (biceps and triceps)

MASTER THE MOVE: Stand with your feet shoulder-width apart and your arms down at your sides. Extend your arms straight behind your body, stretching them back and upward as far as you comfortably can. If your hands reach far enough, clasp them together. Hold for 20 to 30 seconds.

Side Bend

BODY ZONES STRETCHED: mid- and lower back (latissimus dorsi) and side abdominals (obliques)

Without leaning forward, bend at the waist toward the hand on your hip while slowly reaching over your head with the other hand as far as you comfortably can. Hold for 20 to 30 seconds and then stretch the other side.

Bowing Shoulder Stretch

BODY ZONES STRETCHED: mid- and lower back (latissimus dorsi), shoulders (deltoids), and arms (biceps and triceps)

MASTER THE MOVE: Get down on all fours on an exercise mat with your hands and knees about shoulder-width apart. Keep your back flat, your neck straight, and your eyes looking down at the floor. Sit back on your heels, extending your arms out in front of you. Push down slightly with your palms and hold for 20 to 30 seconds.

Cosmetic Nips, Tucks, and Touches

If we all stayed indoors our whole lives and never used our faces to convey emotions by smiling, laughing, or crying, our faces could probably withstand the rigors of age and weather much better than they do.

But that's not reality. We go out into the sunshine, we show our feelings, and the years take their toll. By the time we've reached our thirties or early forties, the first signs of aging have begun to appear, and they show up on every part of our faces. Here's how they develop.

The eyes. Fine lines develop at the sides and underneath the eyes. Puffy upper and lower eyelids may begin to make you seem tired, even when you've been getting your Zzzs. Your eyebrows may seem lower than they once did.

The mouth. Vertical lines develop around your mouth, the corners of which may begin to turn downward in an expression of perpetual unhappiness. Your teeth may look dull, like a dingy wall in need of a fresh coat of paint.

The cheeks. Your cheeks, once full and rosy, may lose their color and their form. Excess skin may seem to drape down from your cheekbones to form jowls. If you've exercised all your life and

kept your weight in check, you may look gaunt: hollow-cheeked, with eyes that seem to sink into your face.

The nose. Your nose may seem larger, its tip thicker and lower than it was in your youth.

The neck. Your neck may begin to look stretched in the center and saggy at the sides, giving you that dreaded turkeylike appearance you may remember from the old ladies in the church choir.

What You Can Do

Granted, those wonderful women from your church were enthusiastic hymn singers and casserole makers. But they weren't sexy, didn't seem athletic, and wouldn't even think of competing on a professional level with younger women or men. In today's world, women lead active lives into their sixties, seventies, and even their eighties. They want their faces and bodies to reflect their youthful outlook on life, says Paul Carniol, M.D., a cosmetic, laser, and reconstructive plastic surgeon in Summit, New Jersey.

A woman whose face looks drawn and wrinkled at 45 can't be magically made to look like a 20-year-old swimsuit model. But she can definitely take steps to make her look like a refreshed, vibrant, energetic woman in her forties. Those steps may include cosmetic surgery, says Dr. Carniol.

"I tell women to think about how they look for their age, how they feel for their age, and what they do at their age," he says. "The best candidates for cosmetic procedures and surgery are those who say, 'I want to look as good as I can for me at my age.' That's achievable."

Where to Begin

A good dermatologist or plastic surgeon will sit down with you to discuss *your* areas of concern and not presume to know what's best for you.

"If a woman were to come in with a frog on her nose, I would still ask, 'What brings you here today?'" says Patricia S. Wexler, M.D., a cosmetic dermatologist in New York City.

Don't let a physician talk you into having your eyelids done if the thing that bothers you most are acne scars that seem more prominent on your cheeks as you age, she counsels.

Here are some ways to make certain that your first trip to the doctor's office is a fruitful one.

Dig into your photo album. A cosmetic consultation isn't like a haircut. Don't bring a picture of Cindy Crawford and ask to be made into her. Instead, select a few photographs of yourself as you've aged: one from your high school years, a few from your twenties, maybe one showing your face in your early thirties. This will help the physician see what elements of your

---

THE PRICE OF BEING CHER

While Cher has admitted to only a few cosmetic procedures, including a rhinoplasty (commonly known as a "nose job"), a breast-lift, and laser removal of two of her tattoos, gossip columnists and tabloids speculate that much more work has been done on that beautiful bod.

Without knowing details, it is difficult to estimate an exact price tag for Cher's new body, but here's a wild guess, based in part on 1997 average surgeon's fees compiled by the American Society of Plastic and Reconstructive Surgeons (ASPRS).

✦ Rhinoplasty	$3,428
✦ Breast-lift	$3,480
✦ Laser tattoo removal	$3,000*
✦ Liposuction	$1,842
✦ Face-lift	$4,783
✦ Abdominoplasty (tummy tuck)	$4,050
✦ Cheek implants	$2,083
GRAND TOTAL	$22,666

*Prices are difficult to estimate for laser tattoo removal. At the Laser and Skin Surgery Center in New York City, sessions cost $300 to $800, but many sessions may be needed, depending on the colors and size of the tattoo, type of ink used, and length of time since the tattoo was done.

---

face may be hiding in the background as you age, says Dr. Carniol.

Talk results. Some patients arrive at the office with a certain procedure (a face-lift, for example) or technology (lasers or ultrasound) in mind. Sometimes, however, a less invasive, less expensive approach would achieve the results you're seeking, notes Dr. Carniol. Focus on the desired result, but ask the physician's opinion about the various ways you could get there.

Interview the physician. Ask how much of the practice is devoted to cosmetic work and how many procedures she has performed. Find out about the physician's training in the newer procedures and whether or not she teaches them to other physicians. Be aware that the before-and-after photos you may be shown reflect best results, not your surgeon's average results, says Dr. Carniol.

Consider cross-specialties. In general, dermatologists are trained to work on the skin, doing procedures such as peels and laser resurfacing and using fillers such as collagen and fat. Plastic surgeons are more associated with face-lifts, brow-lifts, and blepharoplasty (eyelid tucks). In the cosmetic surgery world, however, the barriers have begun to blur. Dermatologists have been among the pioneers of liposuction. Most plastic surgeons have become adept with lasers.

In any case, be sure that your physician is board certified in a relevant field. You can use two reference books found in many public libraries to find board-certified plastic surgeons listed by state and city: *The Directory of Medical Specialists*, published by Marquis Who's Who, and *The Compendium of Certified Medical Specialists*, published by the American Board of Medical Specialties.

Factor the risks. Weighing the risks and benefits of surgery is even more important in cosmetic surgery than in medically necessary operations, since these are procedures simply designed to help you feel better about yourself, not to correct a health problem. Serious complications of anesthesia can be deadly. Infection, scarring, and a temporary or even a permanent loss of feeling are all possible with cosmetic surgery. Your doctor should be

WOMAN TO WOMAN
She Left Her Bags Behind

Jaimie Keyser's friends thought she looked fabulous. After a crushing divorce 5 years before, the Oklahoma City mother of two had dieted and exercised her way into shape, gotten a new hairstyle, and landed a new job. But the beautiful, round, brown eyes that had been her most pronounced feature during her twenties told a story of stress, sun, and genetics. Then, with her 40th birthday approaching, she decided to do something about it.

After my divorce, I knew I had to recover and move on, so I went on a major program to lose weight and tone my body. I also changed the style and color of my hair. My body looked good, and I felt as if I had my soul back. But whenever I checked the mirror, I saw a set of eyes that could have been my mother's. No doubt about it, I looked old.

When I was younger, I had huge, round, brown eyes. People used to comment on them. But as I got older, they just seemed to disappear behind heavy, drooping upper eyelids—just as my mother's had. I had crow's-feet, too. I became more and more self-conscious about my eyes, especially when I went to PTA meetings, where all the other moms looked 25.

Fortunately, I knew I could do something about the situation. After years of managing early childhood education programs, I had decided to change careers and had recently taken a job as a practice coordinator with Dr. Sterling Baker, an ophthalmologic surgeon in Oklahoma City. He specializes in cosmetic surgery, so I would watch all these patients come through the office and leave looking years younger.

Finally, I decided it was my turn.

First, I had Botox for my crow's-feet. Botox is made of

the one to bring these up, and you should sign a form indicating that you understand these risks before undergoing even the most minor cosmetic surgery procedure, says Dr. Carniol.

Make plans. You should leave the physician's office with a stepwise plan that adtoxin from the organisms that cause botulism, a fatal type of food poisoning, but it's very diluted. It temporarily paralyzes and relaxes the muscles around wrinkles. That was really fun to watch. The lines just disappeared.

Then I turned 39, and I had one of those midlife-crisis things. It led to a decision: I really didn't feel old, so I wasn't going to go on looking old. I talked to Dr. Baker and decided to have upper lid blepharoplasties to tighten the skin above my eyes and take out the fat pads at the edges.

The whole procedure took about 45 minutes. I had an IV, and I was put to sleep for about 10 minutes, during which time I got injections to numb the whole area. After that, I was awake and asking questions. There was no pain. All I could feel was tugging.

For that first day, I let my friends take care of me. Mothers hardly ever get babied, so I decided I was going to lie back and enjoy it. They brought me ice packs and I took extra-strength Tylenol. The next day, I was good to go, although I didn't drive for another 24 hours.

The most fun was when I went to church a week later. We're always late, so we came bustling in, and this older woman who was really supportive during my divorce turned around to give me a hug. She said, "You look great today!"

Then I noticed she kept peeking at me all through the service. Afterward, she took my hands and said, "You must love your job and your life, because you are simply glowing!"

Some people thought that I lost weight. And one friend told me, "You have your daughter's eyes." That really meant a lot to me.

I guess there are people who think this is vain. But I think you should make the most of every moment of your life, and to me, looking my best is part of being the best I can be.

Exploring the Possibilities

These days, cosmetic surgery offers a huge array of options to patients who want to appear youthful and more energized. From the top of your forehead down to your neck, there are choices to make about which of your features you want to enhance, how invasive a procedure you'll tolerate, how long a recovery time you can afford, and how much you're interested in spending.

To keep from getting confused or overwhelmed when you're making plans with your surgeon, get to know about some of the possibilities she may suggest before you even get to her office.

Pack your bags. Blepharoplasty is minor surgery to remove excess skin and fat from the upper and lower eyelids. The incision is hidden in the fold of your eyelids. If your vision is impaired because your eyes have become obscured by puffy lids, insurance may pay for this procedure, says Sterling Baker, M.D., an ophthalmologic surgeon in Oklahoma City. The average cost for blepharoplasty of the upper and lower eyelids is about $3,000.

Frown no more. One of the most revolutionary developments in cosmetic rejuvenation in recent years has been the growing popularity of Botox, a highly diluted form of botulinum toxin A. Injected into the deep furrows ("frown lines") of the mid-forehead and crinkly crow's-feet at the edges of your eyes, Botox temporarily paralyzes certain muscle groups that prod facial expressions into wrinkles.

The injections have to be repeated every 4 to

dresses your concerns and reflects the amount of time and money you are willing to spend, says Dr. Carniol. The physician should also explain to you potential complications, recovery times, and care required as you recuperate.

6 months and may cause some bruising. Despite the scary things you may remember about botulism, Botox uses extremely tiny, safe doses. The most serious side effect, says Dr. Wexler, is a drooping of the eyebrow, which is rare. You can expect to pay $400 to $600 per treatment of Botox injections.

Lift a little. Using tools that require minimal incisions, surgeons can reach under the skin to tighten muscles or lift the skin of your forehead, brows, and even the center of the face or neck without subjecting you to the rigors of a full face-lift. In many cases, this may be enough to address your cosmetic concerns. A minimal excision/endoscopic face-lift costs about $5,000.

Lift a lot. A full face-lift, called a rhytidectomy, tightens loose skin from the jowls, jaw, and neck. Scars are hidden around the ear or in the hairline, and the results are often combined with liposuction, laser resurfacing, or both to correct the problems a lift can't help, such as excess fat in the face and neck, surface wrinkles, and blotchy, sun-damaged skin. A traditional face-lift costs about $4,800.

Opt for the big fill. Whereas women once went for extreme face-lifts that pulled their skin up and back so tightly that they looked like they were in a wind tunnel, today's surgeons are responding to calls for a less radical look.

In many cases, that means using fillers to fill in hollowed-out regions of the lower face that have lost their youthful fullness. Generally, these include the deep creases that run between the outer edges of your nostrils to the edges of your lips (the nasolabial folds), perhaps your thinning lips or pinched chin, or the mid to outer cheeks.

REAL-LIFE SCENARIO

She's Going After Liposuction for All the Wrong Reasons

In two weeks, Marguerite is turning 40, and she's going to give herself a birthday present: beautiful legs. She's been telling herself forever that she's going to get rid of the extra padding on her hips and thighs—especially those cellulite dimples—with a strict program of diet and exercise. But Marguerite doesn't take to strict programs of anything very easily, and beach season will be here before she knows it. She's already purchased a gorgeous new bandeau she wants to show off, but she absolutely will not wear it if her legs aren't perfect, especially in front of her husband, who she fears is losing interest in her. So she's off to the plastic surgeon to get those dimples vacuumed away through liposuction. All the stars do it. Why shouldn't she? It's as easy as one-two-three. Or is it?

Marguerite is off to a great start with her diet and exercise program, and if she sticks with it, she'll definitely improve her look. But for several reasons, she isn't the kind of liposuction candidate that most surgeons like to treat.

Chronically overweight people are not likely to achieve wonderful and permanent results, simply because their

"A lift lifts. It doesn't fill," says Dr. Wexler, who often uses fillers to restore fullness to the cheeks.

When it comes to fillers, the choice is ever widening. Dr. Wexler often selects the safest, simplest alternative: the patient's own fat. For this, she performs a two-in-one procedure that liposuctions a woman's own fat from her hips, thighs, or abdomen and uses a bit of it to fill areas that could use a little plumping up.

What can't be used at once is frozen securely for monthly injections. After a year of treatments, Dr. Wexler guarantees 30 percent of the injected fat will remain permanently, which is almost always enough to fill grooves and pits. The weight is likely to soar after the procedure, and the fat will come back—usually in nearby areas, although it may return even to areas previously liposuctioned. The worst candidates are those whose weight yo-yos.

Marguerite has another problem: She has a hard time following strict programs. Liposuction is a surgical procedure that demands strict adherence to a doctor's orders, before, during, and after the surgery. Not doing so could compromise Marguerite's health.

Marguerite may also be unhappy with the results. Liposuction can smooth stubborn lumps of fat and provide a nicer contour to the figure, but it's not always effective at getting rid of cellulite, which is a normal and natural phenomenon in women over 30.

The biggest flashing "error" light in Marguerite's story, though, is her hope that liposuction may reignite her husband's interest in her. Removing fat off her thighs will not give her a happy life. At best, it will give her self-image a little boost.

Expert consulted
Patricia S. Wexler, M.D.
Cosmetic dermatologist
New York City

average price for an office visit for fat injections in the face and neck is about $1,000.

Get cheeky. Ironically, it is often the women who stayed in the best shape throughout their youth who suffer the ravages of age earliest, says Dr. Wexler. That's because as we age, muscle tone and fat are lost in the face, and the skin doesn't retract but hangs on the facial bones like a half-dismantled tent sagging from its poles.

When more bulk is needed, physicians turn to a variety of products, many of which can be cut or rolled to fit the depression to be filled. Gore-Tex makes one such material; another is Allo-Derm, a natural product derived from sterilized human skin cells treated to remove all cells that would transmit disease, leaving only the structural network of skin.

AlloDerm can be rolled to fill lips or folded over to level out an acne or chicken pox scar. One form of Gore-Tex comes in threads to fill a long wrinkle line. Other fillers are derived from bovine (cow) collagen or collagen grown from samples of your own tissue in a special processing laboratory. The cost of fillers and their placement varies widely. Collagen injections cost an average of $325 per site.

Peel away the years. Physicians or aestheticians (skin specialists trained to perform some of the less-involved procedures such as laser hair removal or light chemical peels) may recommend that you have a chemical peel, which comes in many forms. Glycolic acid, trichloracetic acid (TCA), salicylic acid, and phenol peels are applied to the face and perhaps the neck, chest, and hands for a brief period of time. Fans, ice packs, and sometimes local anesthesia will be used to reduce the immediate irritation; your skin will crust and then peel over the ensuing days to give you a smoother skin surface. The average charge for a chemical peel is $1,600.

Laser those lines. Entranced by *Star Wars* and planetarium light shows, many women believe laser beams are virtually magic, able to blaze through a person's wrinkles in a flash, without going through the trauma of plastic surgery.

The truth is that lasers come in many different forms. The Erbium-YAG laser can smooth fine wrinkles close to the skin's surface and even out irregular skin tones, producing results similar to those of a medium-strength peel. The more powerful carbon dioxide laser can erase deeper wrinkles and photodamage, but at a price. The burn left by such a laser takes weeks to heal, and the redness that follows can last up to a year. Full-face laser resurfacing costs about $2,800.

Go lightly. A new technique, microdermabrasion, has recently arrived on the American cosmetic scene from Europe. Known by such names as the Parisian Peel, Power Peel, and Derma Peel, this is a way to gently buff the skin with a machine that blows purified abrasive particles against it, then vacuums them away. Virtually painless, microdermabrasion can be performed quickly and without anesthesia. You'll be a bit pink, but you can return to work or your normal activities immediately. A series of five or more sessions is generally performed on a weekly or biweekly basis, followed up with monthly sessions. Microdermabrasion costs vary. You can expect to pay $100 to $200 a treatment.

Farther South

Aging doesn't stop at the face, of course, and sometimes the aging problems that most affect our appearance are well south of the chin. Cosmetic surgeons can also help you in those areas.

Sculpt your curves. Has your bikini spent the last decade stuffed deep in your pajama drawer? Even with exercise and a healthy eating style, most women notice that their weight begins to settle in problem areas as they approach middle age. Liposuction can help to smooth stubborn bulges in your hips, upper thighs, flanks, abdomen, and upper back.

"Liposuction won't replace weight loss, but it will contour you. It will give you back your curves," says Dr. Carniol. "It can significantly improve the contours of people who are moderately overweight and have not been able to lose weight through diet and exercise."

You should seek out an experienced liposuction surgeon who aims for a three-dimensional, whole-body approach. Otherwise, if you gain weight, it will settle in areas you didn't have liposuctioned, says Dr. Carniol. Liposuction of a single body area costs about $1,800.

Erase your spider veins. Even if your legs are in great shape, you may be reluctant to wear shorts because of tiny red or purple lines lying close to the surface of the skin. A physician can inject these with a special solution to make them fade, in a procedure called sclerotherapy.

The process will require you to wear support stockings even after your dressings have been removed. Sclerotherapy costs an average of $300. Some physicians are using special lasers to target the pigment in spider veins; this will probably cost more, closer to the $500 range.

Recapture Your Smile

You're not a smoker and you brush, floss, use mouthwash, and see the dentist twice a year. So why the dingy smile?

"Teeth will darken with aging," sympathizes Stephen H. Fassman, D.D.S., a dentist and attending surgeon at the New York University Medical Center in New York City.

To brighten your smile again, you may want to consider bleaching your teeth. If you do, here's the way to go about it.

Skip the drugstore. No matter what they claim, companies aren't allowed to sell over-the-counter products strong enough to significantly whiten teeth, says Dr. Fassman. True teeth-bleaching formulas are considered drugs by the Food and Drug Administration. They have to be dispensed by a dentist, he says.

Start fast. In a single visit, your dentist can paint a bleach on your teeth that will lighten your teeth by a half to one full shade.

Bleach at home. You'll be fitted with soft plastic mouth guards that fit over your teeth, top and bottom. For 1 to 2 hours a night for 2 to 4 weeks, you'll fill the guard with a white, sticky gel that you get from your dentist and fit the guard snugly over your teeth.

"Within a few days, the change will be very apparent. Your teeth should be at least three shades lighter by the end of the second week," Dr. Fassman says.

"At-home bleaching is usually the method of choice," says Dr. Fassman, "but some people like to combine an in-office bleaching with the gel you use at home." The total cost for whitening your teeth will be $450 to $1,000, depending on the methods you use.

Making Your Decision

So now that you know the possibilities, how will you choose the ones that are right for you? Here are some factors to consider.

Mix and match. You may find that you can't meet your needs with just one procedure. Often, a combination of approaches is more effective, says Dee Anna Glaser, M.D., assistant professor of dermatology at St. Louis University. She weighs many factors when it comes to deciding which approaches to use on a woman's aging face.

If your deepest lines run vertically over your upper lip, you may want to consider having a laser treatment just there and using a medium-strength TCA peel on the rest of your face and neck to even out your skin tone and give you a smooth, bright, and youthful appearance, Dr. Glaser says.

High and low maintenance. A peel requires care during phases of oozing and crusting. "Some women are going to be grossed out or don't want to follow a lot of instructions," she says. For them, a laser rejuvenation may be best, even though the healing time is longer, since a synthetic dressing is applied to the entire face afterward and a nurse changes it in the office.

Putting aside time. A laser resurfacing procedure generally requires 2 full weeks of recuperation, during which you won't want to be seen in public. Many plastic surgery procedures also require hefty amounts of time spent "lying low" as bruises and scars heal enough to be covered with camouflage makeup. Some women would rather commit to numerous small procedures such as microdermabrasion, Botox injections, or light peels until their lives slow down enough to consider a more dramatic step. Others want to have everything done at once. "They might want to get it all done quickly in time for a daughter's wedding," Dr. Glaser says.

What you can afford. A face-lift, upper and lower blepharoplasties, and a full-face laser resurfacing with a peel of the neck, chest, and hands would make Grandma Moses look like a glowing beauty. But they would add up to almost $12,000.

"Before you do anything, ask yourself, 'What do I really want? What's really going to make me feel better?'" suggests Dr. Carniol. It may be that cosmetic surgery will give you a rejuvenated look that is well worth the price. On the other hand, it may turn out that what you really want is a relaxing cruise in the Mediterranean.

Winning the Battle of the Mane

Good cuts, bad color, strange or expensive products—most of us have lived through a whole gamut of experiences during our quest for the perfect 'do. Then, just when we thought we'd won the battle, our hair started to change. During or just after our thirties, "the grays" began their assault. To make matters worse, our hair started growing more slowly and becoming finer.

So now what?

So now it's time to update the 'do, to give it back the shine, resiliency, color, and shape that looked so great just a few short years ago.

Finding Your New Look

Every woman feels a little anxiety, as well as a little excitement, when she's on the verge of changing her hairstyle. And for no small reason. She may enter the salon as one person and come out looking like someone else altogether. People will react to her a little differently than they ever have before. And when she looks in the mirror, she'll meet a new person, whom she hopes she'll like.

It can end up being a very good experience or a very bad one. Here are some ways to tilt the odds in your favor.

Assess from head to toe. Your hair is part of a package, so selecting a style that suits only your face can undermine your entire look. Not only should you consider the shape of your face, but also your height, weight, what your day-to-day life is like, and how handy or not you are with styling, says Victoria Meekins, vice president of Kenneth's Salon/KEB Associates at the Waldorf-Astoria Hotel in New York City. The key to a great look is homing in on the styles that best suit the total you.

Be open to change. Committing to a hairstyle isn't like taking an oath of allegiance. "It's only hair; it'll always grow back," says stylist Alex Ioannou, co-owner of Trio Salon in Chicago. On average, hair grows ½ inch a month. So experiment, try new things. If it doesn't work, there's always next time.

Define yourself. Even a hairdresser who knows you well isn't psychic. Without specific examples, she may not understand what you mean by an updated or youthful new hairstyle.

"What you think is attractive and what I

think is attractive may be two very different things," says Keith Ayotte, creative director for Vidal Sassoon in Atlanta.

So give the subject some thought *before* you see a stylist.

Collect images. Whenever you see a picture of a model with a hairstyle that you like, tear it out. Start a collection. Don't worry about whether any of the styles will look good on you. "Pictures give me a better idea of what you're looking for. Making the style work is my job," explains Ayotte.

Building a Better Partnership

On-the-job experience and constant training help professional stylists develop a keen sense of what's right—or wrong—for a client. Your role in this transaction isn't passive. Whether you've seen the same stylist for decades or you're searching for someone new to help you update your look, there are steps stylists say that you can take to ease the process.

Book a consultation. You don't have to get your hair cut and styled every time you step into a salon. It'll probably feel weird walking out without a cut, but getting an expert opinion is a great first step to giving your image a fresh new edge.

Fire a warning shot. When you're ready for an update, put your hairdresser on alert. Call a couple of days before your appointment and tell the pro that you want to try something new. Your stylist will probably be excited by this creative opportunity and love the idea of having the time to research some great options.

Pick and choose. There are many different types of salons. Go to one that caters to contemporary style without being too avant-garde. The people at the modern salon are more grounded. They are the ones who know how to make a trend wearable.

Shop with care. Look for an experienced stylist. If in doubt, a salon receptionist can offer background on the stylist that you're thinking about visiting.

Build a relationship. Once you've chosen a stylist, stick with her. Someone who knows you will be much better at advising you than a complete stranger would be. Whenever you become

A good stylist can direct attention away from problem areas merely by changing the shape of your hair, according to Frank Shipman, owner and stylist at Technicolor Salon and Day Spa in Allentown, Pennsylvania. "Weight lines," which establish strong horizontal "edges," can do wonders. A weight line is the place on your hairstyle that draws attention and appears to have the most visual weight or volume.

A weight line can add definition to your face. Consider, for example, a jawline that's softened by a double chin. To remedy this problem, one option is a bob that's slightly raised in the back. Another option is putting more visual weight near the temple to give the illusion of a narrower jaw.

Another great use of a weight line is in deflecting attention from a less-than-perfect neck. In this case, shift the weight line higher so that the thicker hair is closer to the crown, drawing attention away from your neck.

bored with your current cut and color, she'll be your best ally in choosing a new look. And you'll know that you can trust her judgment.

Do's and Don'ts

We live in an era of fashion flexibility. You can go long or short, curly or straight without incurring the wrath of the fashion police. Yet it's still possible to end up with a "don't" when you're updating a 'do. Here are some suggestions to keep you on the right track.

Be true to you. "I don't think that sticking with the latest trend is what makes you look younger," says Ayotte. It's fine to pay attention to the popular length, style, and color, yet these shouldn't dictate your choices. Regardless of the look that others are touting, go with what works for you. "You'll look beautiful, and when you look

beautiful, you'll look and feel younger," he says.

Cut the curl. Meekins spent the 1960s with her locks wrapped in juice cans, and the 1970s using chemical straighteners. No matter what this New York City resident tried, controlling her frizzy hair was a struggle, so she went natural. Doing her hair became easier, but there was something about her look that she just didn't like.

Finally, she asked her stylist about it. The candid answer was an eye-opener, "Your tight, short curls make you look old." Taking her cue from the expert, she grew her hair almost to her shoulders and started straightening it again. But this time she's getting a professional blow-dry styling every 3 to 4 days, instead of chemical treatments.

Try longer locks. It's tempting to solve an image dilemma by cutting off your hair. In fact, some women think that chopping their locks is a rite of passage. "It drives me crazy that so many women buy into the myth that they have to go shorter as they get older," says salon owner and stylist Frank Shipman of Technicolor Salon and Day Spa in Allentown, Pennsylvania. "Shoulder-length hair can look fabulous if it suits you."

Accept your hair. Long, short, thick, thin, straight, curly—whatever your hair's characteristics—it's more than likely that you want to change something about it. But the grass isn't always greener on the other side of the salon. Find a style that works with your hair's texture and growth patterns. You'll be happier with the result. Ioannou says that working with, rather than against, your hair eliminates the passé habits of setting, spraying, and teasing.

Hairstyles That Complement Glasses

First came the shock of discovering that you need bifocals—or that your eyes have weakened over the past year. Now you have to sort through a huge array of eyeglass frames to find a shape that works with your hair, the shape of your face, and your personality.

Ayotte explains where to start.

Balance the act. The main consideration is balancing the volume and shape of your eyeglasses with your hairstyle. Identify the strongest elements of your hairstyle and then choose a frame that matches.

Combine classics. A classic hairstyle, one that needs minimal styling and is one length all over the head, is best suited to frame shapes that have also stood the test of time. Simple round or square eyeglasses are good options.

Measure the extreme. A strong, trendy style demands eyeglasses that can hold their own. For example, bangs that are little more than a high fringe require eyeglasses with strong lines. Ovals, squares with triangular edges, even the good old cat's-eyes, like the ones you might have worn as a kid, work wonders.

Pull back your hair. A classic chignon or ponytail at the nape of the neck gives you many choices for eyeglass frames. Merely choose a style that suits the shape of your face.

Repeat the geometry. Continue the circular motifs of curly hair in your eyeglasses. Round or oval frames look beautiful. Square frames, on the other hand, are too much of a contrast. Since even short curly hair has movement, choose frames that don't have a lot of detail.

Show your face. Large eyeglasses cover quite a bit of the face. This isn't a problem, as long as you keep your hair under control. Otherwise, people will ask, "Who's hiding behind those glasses and all that hair?" One simple step is cutting off long bangs.

Colorful Options

All our lives we've been led to believe that gray hair marks the end of our youth. By our early thirties, we're diligently seeking and plucking those harbingers of "old age" and worrying about what's around the corner. True, some of us look on those first few grays as a badge of honor. But over time, concern mounts as more and more appear.

As we age, the cells in our hair produce less pigment, explains Ivan Cohen, M.D., associate professor of dermatology at Yale University School of Dermatology. First, the hair shifts to a lighter color, then to gray, and then on to white. This process varies—and sometimes stalls—depending on your genetic heritage.

Sooner or later we all start wondering if it's time to add color. This isn't an all-or-nothing decision. In fact, most women ease into the process with a variety of subtler treatments: demi- or semi-permanent color, highlights, lowlights, blending, foils. The greatest thing about color is that you can always change it, although you can never take it back to natural.

Blend away the gray. You've probably already seen foils in action at your favorite salon. Women receiving this treatment have clumps of hair sticking out at all angles, with what looks like strips of aluminum foil wrapped around the base of each section. Don't laugh—remember how we used to look in skullcaps, with thin strands of hair sticking out everywhere? Foils don't jab at our scalp like the "crochet" hooks did.

Rather than applying color to single strands, foils add color to larger groupings. Color is closer to the base, so touch-ups aren't as frequent, and there's more control over the color placement. According to Meekins, foils also allow the colorist to apply two, three, sometimes even four colors to the hair for a more natural effect.

Face reality. Reverting to the color of your teens and twenties is a mistake. Your skin color has lightened, so you may not be able to carry the stronger color. Use it only as a reference point for going one or two levels lighter, suggests Shipman. Also keep in mind that warm hair colors are usually more flattering. The tones reflect on the face to give it a glow, rather than washing out the complexion as cool colors tend to do.

Go for broke. When it's time to take the plunge into total coverage, consider the benefits. You'll have softer, shinier hair that gives your face a glow. "Allover color isn't a horrible thing. It can be really quite an esthetic experience," says Shipman.

Remember your past. Highlights and lowlights give the illusion of more shape and a youthful appearance, says Meekins. The sun-kissed color that your hair turned during the summers of your youth suggests wonderful highlights for your current hair.

Shine on. If you're still debating the merits of coloring your gray, consider the hidden benefits, Meekins suggests. Color processes add body, dimension, shine, softness, and texture—all the things that are missing in gray hair.

Try a teaser. When the gray strands first appear, try using processes that cover gray rather than remove pigment from the hair. You won't get total coverage, but the gray is camouflaged. It now blends into your natural color. A semi- or demi-permanent does just that, depositing color on the hair. At first, you might just want to add a bit of color to brighten the base. "This is kind of like a tease, to ease you into permanent hair-coloring processes," Ayotte says.

Graying Gracefully

Coloring your hair isn't the only way to reenergize your appearance, especially if gray or white hair is the perfect color for the lighter complexion you've gained in recent years. This doesn't mean that you're doomed to looking older than you feel. Shiny, healthy gray or white hair can make you appear full of vitality.

Blue clues. The yellow cast and dullness that affect gray or silver hair can be washed right out of your hair. Meekins says that shampoos with a violet or blue base maintain your hair's vibrancy and clarity.

Use protein. Conditioners with protein and vitamins add instant volume to your tresses. Hair absorbs protein, then swells so that it looks thicker. The effect won't last forever, says Meekins, but it's a wonderful way to add volume. Spritzers and other styling products that include keratin, which is a protein, give strength and shine. Keratin also helps with the breakage problem that crops up with processed hair, she adds.

Products with silicone bases also give your hair shine, but not as much as keratin. You might also want to consider a salon application of glosses and intensifiers.

Wash 'n' wear with care. Brush, shampoo, and wash your hair gently. Wet hair is fragile. Towel it dry carefully, and brush it without tugging. It's preferable to use a brush with bristles that don't have sharp ends. Meekins suggests that when your hair is dry and you head out the door, put on a hat, wrap a scarf over your hair, or keep to the shade.

WOMAN TO WOMAN
She Jumped Off the Chemical Seesaw

Valerie Hoffman, a lawyer in Chicago, started to gray during her college years. She loved the effect when she was young, but as her other features matured, she thought that coloring her shoulder-length hair might give her a younger look. It took a great haircut and re-verting to her natural, white hair for Valerie to discover that long, colored hair wasn't her path to the fountain of youth.

When I was growing up, my hair had always been a light brown color, but when I went to college, it started turning gray. What a surprise that was! I actually liked the effect, and when I became a lawyer, the mature look that it gave me helped to foster my clients' trust in me.

By the time I reached 28, however, I started to feel that I was looking too old for my age. Naturally, I figured that dyeing my hair back to its original color would help. Unfortunately, my hair wasn't willing to go along with the plan.

Every 6 weeks, I'd go to my stylist to dye it. But in between appointments, I would spend a lot of time playing outdoor sports, and the exposure to the sun would fade the brown to a washed-out blonde color. The changes were obvious and not at all flattering.

It was no use. It was time to stop the dye jobs and I wanted a quick transition that didn't involve stripping out the color. My stylist convinced me that the way to do that was to cut my hair very, very short.

It was a scary suggestion. I love long hair, and I was afraid I'd end up looking like a boy. But I hated the coloring so much that my decision was clear-cut. When my stylist was finished with me, my hair was about an inch long.

How did I feel when I looked into the mirror?

My hair looked fabulous, and now at age 45, it still does. Its length and pure white color are a great combination. I no longer look dowdy, and my small features don't disappear under a mop of hair.

All in all, I'm really happy with my look now. And I wish the same for other women. Take the bold step—it can make a huge difference.

Color Me Youthful

Back in the early 1980s, you could walk into almost any clothing shop and find a woman scouring the racks for colors that matched her "season." It was the era of color revolution in fashion, launched almost single-handedly by a book called *Color Me Beautiful*.

That book brought color theory to the masses, showing how wearing the right colors can make anyone look fabulous. By assessing skin undertones, a reader could categorize herself as a winter, spring, summer, or autumn color type, and then learn to use image-enhancing hues to her best advantage.

The concept is sound. Color can bring energy and vitality to your appearance. And once you know how, you can apply the concept to your entire wardrobe.

Compliments of the Season

If you've ever "had your colors done," as the expression goes, then you already know that using the right colors near your face is like getting an instant face-lift and chemical peel all in one. But if the colors you're wearing aren't flat-tering, any imperfections you may have are going to be magnified. Even in shorts, the wrong color will emphasize skin flaws on your legs.

In *Color Me Beautiful*, author Carole Jackson categorized people into four groups, named after the seasons and based on an assessment of skin undertones, hair color, and eye color. Each season has a palette of colors that suit it. Think of the dominant colors in each season of the year, and you'll have a good idea of which colors belong to its group.

It's a model that image consultants like Donna Fujii, who trains beauty consultants in San Francisco and Tokyo, follow to this day, although many have created subcategories within the seasons and developed new groups. Her award-winning book, *Color with Style*, expanded color theory to embrace the diversity of skin tones for African-American, Asian, and Hispanic women.

If you haven't already, take the time to read both books. They're great primers for doing your colors. But if you want to start right now, here are some tips from Fujii and other fashion experts that will point you in the right direction.

Identify your undertone. Even experts use a trial-and-error method. Pieces of fabric from each season are draped around the client's neck, one at a time. If the skin looks washed out or sallow, the color is wrong. After several colors are tested, a pattern becomes clear. Skin that has blue undertones (summer and winter) looks best in cool colors; so orange-yellow fabrics aren't flattering. Skin with yellow undertones (spring and autumn) needs warm colors. Vibrant blue-violet, for example, brings out the worst.

As you assess your skin, keep in mind that the coolness or warmth of skin tones has nothing to do with the light or dark quality. Darker skins do tend to be warmer, but this isn't a hard-and-fast rule.

Check the contrast. It's not enough to know if you can wear warm or cool colors. The contrast between hair and skin is also a consideration. High-contrast women—brunettes with fair skin, for example—can wear stronger colors, whereas women with gray or salt-and-pepper hair are low-contrast and need to tone things down. A low-contrast person can, however, get away with stronger colors in evening light.

Lower the contrast. Having your colors done isn't a one-time event. As we age, our hair and skin lighten or dull, so the color value and intensity that we can wear may soften a notch or two. If, for example, you usually wear black and other dark colors, charcoal gray and winter white may now be more suit-

COLORS THAT HIDE

You can use the colors in your wardrobe to get thinner instantly.

Stop laughing. It's true.

It's simply a matter of optical illusion, of drawing attention to your assets and away from your liabilities. In wardrobe color theory, it's called color blocking, and whether you realize it or not, you already know the basics, says Jan Larkey, an image consultant in Pittsburgh and author of *Flatter Your Figure*.

Every time you combine separates you're working with color blocking. When you try on a dark blouse with pastel slacks, for example, you instinctively know something is wrong. You look off-balance because, visually, light colors make areas look larger while dark colors have the opposite effect.

To fix the imbalance, all you have to do is put on a jacket or sweater of the same color as the pants. Now there's proportionally less of the dark color visible. The one-color silhouette creates a long, tall vertical, and, if you leave the jacket or sweater open, the lapels form two more slimming vertical lines down the center front.

Any outfit in a single, darker color takes off pounds. Don't sabotage the effect by adding a belt in a contrasting color that chops you in half. Shift the contrast higher—to a yoke on a blouse, for example—and voilà!—instantly wider shoulders. This is a great way to balance a larger lower body. Shift the contrast to a color band around the hips, on the other hand, and you're in trouble, unless you have a small derriere and hips.

To develop a keen sense of color blocking, start by honestly assessing your body. Create vertical color blocks over any body parts you wish were taller or slimmer, and horizontal color blocks on the parts you wish were wider. Now make a point of never placing colors in a manner that draws attention to trouble spots. When all else fails, you can create a winning look by combining medium-color separates with a flattering scarf at the neck.

IS BASIC BLACK FOR EVERYONE?

Colors go in and out of fashion, but like an old, steadfast friend, black is always there for you. Sometimes it steps aside for brown or blue among your wardrobe basics, but no other color switches from serious business to casual daytime to evening wear so effortlessly.

Unfortunately, there's a problem: Few women look good with black next to their faces. Hardly any of us can pull off the stunning effect that black creates on a silver-haired woman who has taken the time to define her eyebrows and apply a strong lipstick color. But does this mean we have to give up all the black hanging in our closets? Not at all.

In her book *Quickstyle: How to Expand, Enhance, and Update Your Wardrobe with Accessories*, fashion guru Christine Kunzelman espouses the tremendous benefits of wearing a basic black collarless dress but suggests adding accessories and layering it over with other clothes.

Her idea is to place your most appealing colors nearest your face. Consider downplaying black with color in a loose-buttoned overblouse, an open or closed jacket, a turtleneck underneath a black collarless garment, a sweater draped over the shoulders with the sleeves tied together in front, or a scarf.

Combine your colors with care, however, as your choices can pack on the years. For the most up-to-date look, mix black with brown, khaki, or other neutrals.

black is beautiful, brown looks dowdy. A year later the entire scene can totally reverse. Don't take trends too seriously, says Fujii. Study them, use what appeals to you, then find your own way. Here's some advice to help you.

Remain neutral. For your clothes, combine neutrals. Dress simply and spice up the look with interesting shoes, says image consultant Diana Kilgour of Vancouver, Canada. In any case, it's a good idea to keep your shoes current.

Oust the old combos. Seek out interesting new ways to combine your separates and accessories, suggests Kilgour. A continental, European effect might mix winter and summer colors, mix neutrals, or add baby blue, black, brown, or charcoal to navy blue. For a suit, combine black and brown rather than black and emerald green.

Pick and choose. "In every trend—in every season—there's going to be more than one color palette," says Fujii. Home in on the colors that work for you. Pick three, maybe four, but never more than five. Even within a single color trend, there's a range of tones, so you should be able to find one that works with your complexion.

Context counts. The environment in which you plan to wear an outfit is just as important as color suitability. For example, if you're wearing peach and people around you are in black, you'll look too young, says Kilgour. So plan ahead and try to fit in with the crowd.

able. Salt-and-pepper hair might look better in sand, taupe, or pearl gray.

"I'm wearing colors today that I couldn't wear several years ago," says 49-year-old image consultant Pat Newquist, owner of Wardrobe Image in Tempe, Arizona. To be safe, consult an expert every 5 years.

On the Edge of Trends

Every few months, there is a flurry of activity as designers and fashion experts announce the season's colors: bright pink is in, pastels are out;

Face Up to Colors

Our natural skin tones, hair color, and clothes aren't the only colorful things about us, of course. We also wear makeup. And where enhancing our facial features is concerned, it's tough to let go of old habits. In fact, most of us tend to wear makeup the same way for 10, even 20 years, says Newquist.

When we do this, we're walking away from a wonderful opportunity. With new application methods, colors, and products, we can shed years. In fact, makeup expert Linda Stasi of New York City, former beauty editor and columnist for *Cosmopolitan*, *Elle*, and *New Woman* magazines and coauthor of *Boomer Babes: A Woman's Guide to the New Middle Ages* says that the effect of reworking eyebrows is as dramatic as a face-lift.

Pat Newquist, Linda Stasi, and Donna Fujii, who has her own line of makeup and skin treatments, offer more advice.

Correct and conceal. Dark circles under the eyes need a color corrector and a concealer. Apply the corrector first. The color you select depends on your skin tones. Although there are huge color variations within ethnic groups, you can narrow your color choice by considering your background. African-Americans can choose yellow or amber, Asian skin needs pink, Mediterranean is best suited to yellow, and Scandinavian selects a whitish product. Blend the edges of the corrector, then apply concealer that is almost the same color as your skin.

Go lightly. Skin tones lighten or dull with age, so it makes sense to go a little lighter on the makeup. Use colors that aren't as intense as those you used before. For example, shift from black to brown eyeliner. Choose soft, sheer makeup that's blended with brushes rather than your fingertips. Ensure that the color doesn't sit on top of your skin, and wear neutral eye shadow. Your blush should match the color that your cheeks get when you're working out. Apply blush below the cheekbones.

Update regularly. Lipstick may last a year or more, but it's still a good idea to reevaluate your makeup colors at least once a year. What you see may inspire you to make a bold change, drop the eyeliner, or buy a new lipstick that's a few shades lighter or darker than the one you're using. Splurge. After all, lipstick costs less than dinner and a movie.

Dressed to Impress

The wish: You walk into a party, and the room lights up. Everyone is smiling in your direction. You look fabulously youthful, vibrant, stylish. People are happy just to be with you.

The fear: You walk into a party and people cover their eyes and mouths to hide their embarrassed looks and snickers. You look outlandish or silly in clothing that's too young or too wild for you.

The reality: You walk into a party and nobody notices. You look the same as you always have because you're afraid to wear a style that's new or different.

Nothing can take years off your look faster than the right clothes, but changing the way you dress is risky business. We're all a little afraid of making fashion mistakes. So we end up dressing as we always dressed and dating ourselves a little bit at a time.

The great news is that there's really no need to be so timid. In fact, with a little bit of knowledge and a few tricks up your sleeve, you can "loosen up your look" (that's image consultant lingo for dressing in a more youthful way) and

turn your wish into reality, while leaving your fear behind you.

Avoid Wearing the Right Things the Wrong Way

So many department stores and so little time. Where do you begin?

Tips from image consultant Pat Newquist, owner of Wardrobe Image in Tempe, Arizona, will help you hunt for the silhouettes, garments, and accessories that instantly update a wardrobe.

Evolve gradually. Like a big-game hunter, use a cautious approach. Newquist often tells clients of her 16-year-old company, "If you don't know how to wear it, you'll look too young." At first, stick to classics and add only a few trendy items. Proceed one step at a time. That way, even if you make a mistake, it will be a small one.

Spot the trends. A great way to dress for a youthful look is to pay attention to what's hot, says Newquist. But it takes a bit of work to identify worthwhile trends. The best place to start is in the fashion magazines. What are the models wearing? Notice details of color and cut. What styles do you think might look good on you?

Also pay close attention to ads and watch what the stars are wearing on the fashion, music, and movie awards shows. These people are in the business of keeping an up-to-date, attractive image.

Study brands. Look for labels that create a womanly interpretation of junior trends. For example, a few years ago, the younger crowd was wearing fitted, waist-length leather jackets. Designer Dana Buchman offered her customers leather jackets that still looked fitted but weren't quite as tight and had lower hemlines than clothes made for young women.

Shopping Savvy

Developing a flattering, age-defying collection of clothing starts with careful shopping. Newquist gives her clients specific guidelines to follow when they're ready to hit the stores.

Dress up. "When you plan to try on clothes, get dressed up really nice," says Newquist. Wear good-looking undergarments and slip on brand-new panty hose so that you're more comfortable with the image staring back at you.

Window-shop. Spend a weekend browsing through clothing stores. Don't take any money, just try things on. It's important to go alone so that you're free of influence from others. Be playful: Try on whatever catches your fancy.

Fit loose. "It's better to wear your clothes

SHOES THAT SHINE

Both by the way they look and the way they feel, a pair of shoes can either age you or put a youthful spring in your step. Once you own a pair of classic pumps and flats in your basic wardrobe color, you can start exploring some other options.

Accessory guru Christine Kunzelman writes in her book *Quickstyle: How to Expand, Enhance, and Update Your Wardrobe with Accessories* that every wardrobe should include ankle boots, ballet flats, colored tennis shoes, espadrilles, lace-up brogues, loafers, riding boots, spectator pumps, strappy high heels, and strappy leather sandals.

Pat Newquist, owner of Wardrobe Image in Tempe, Arizona, says it's also very important to keep your shoes current. Just buying one or two up-to-date styles every season gives your wardrobe a fashion edge. Shoe stores are so full of eye candy that you're certain to home in on footwear that works with your updated image.

But remember: It's hard to project an energetic attitude when your tootsies are aching, so to make sure you get a good fit, follow this advice.

- ❥ Feet grow with age; have yours measured regularly.
- ❥ Measure both feet and fit the largest.
- ❥ Allow ⅜ to ½ inch of space between the end of the shoe and your longest toe.
- ❥ Accept only a minimum amount of slippage at the heels.
- ❥ When you're trying on shoes, position the ball of your foot in the widest part (ball pocket) of the shoe.

---

loose rather than snug," says Newquist. "They'll make you look 10 to 20 pounds thinner. You should be able to insert two fingers into a waistband. Pants and skirts are too small through the hips if you can't pinch out 2 inches of fabric."

The Wrinkle Check

Your face stares back at you from the mirror, and for the umpteenth time this week, you see that new wrinkle at the corner of your mouth.

Scrutinizing your face while applying makeup is a rite of passage that we all go through. But there's a whole other set of wrinkles, not on our face, that age us and are visible from many feet away from the mirror.

The next time that you dress, look for diagonal, horizontal, and vertical wrinkles. These, says international fit and sewing expert Sandra Betzina, point to fit problems. Host of the television show *Sew Perfect* on the cable channel Home and Garden Television and author of the *Power Sewing* book series, Betzina gives thousands of women advice and guidance on garment fit.

Rounded back pulls up front neckline

Narrow upper chest doesn't fill out front

Protruding tummy pulls up front hem

Forward-pitched, sloping, or uneven shoulders. Diagonal wrinkles travel across the shoulders and neck. Try shoulder pads, says Jan Larkey, an image consultant in Pittsburgh and author of *Flatter Your Figure*. Place the blunt end of the pad just beyond your sleeve seam to hide rounded shoulders. If one shoulder is higher than the other, use a thinner pad on that side of the garment. Larkey pushes her own pads toward the back to compensate for a curved spine.

Full high hips. There are small horizontal wrinkles immediately under the front and back waistband. Wear garments that hang from the widest part of your lower body, particularly if your hip fullness starts almost immediately below the waist.

Makeup is part of the problem. A consultant can show Andrea how to choose and apply subtle, attractive colors. As for her hair, she should shift the ponytail to the base of the neck and twist it into a chignon.

Her pleated skirt can work in her favor, so long as it fits properly. Pleats should hang straight, without opening, so if Andrea's skirt is fluffing at the hip, there's a problem.

The tight sweater and ankle socks are big mistakes. Clothing that reveals your figure is wrong for the office at any age, and ankle socks with a skirt and business shoes are always inappropriate.

Andrea's overall look, particularly the sweater, is more "social casual," than "business casual," which means it would be appropriate only on "Casual Friday." Even then, a better option is a twinset (jewel neckline pullover and matching cardigan) paired with tailored slacks.

Expert consulted
Jan Larkey
Image consultant
Author of Flatter Your Figure
Pittsburgh

Full upper arms. Diagonal wrinkles cross the upper arm near the shoulders and grow steeper along the lower arm. Some well-known designers insert a vertical seam along the top of the sleeve. It can be let out for nicer fit.

Low or flat bottom. "Frowning" horizontal wrinkles form under the back crotch, and the pants' waist pulls down at the center back. Invest in body-shaping undergarments that lift a low bottom or pad a flat derriere.

Narrow upper chest. The shoulder seams drop off the shoulder, and there are horizontal wrinkles across the upper chest. This figure problem is very difficult to fit in ready-to-wear garments. The best solution is to hire a dressmaker.

Protruding tummy. Side seams pull forward, skirts hike up at center front, and pants are tight through the crotch. Waist darts emphasize your roundness. Instead, choose garments that hang straight from the fullest part of the tummy. Look for hidden tummy panels that control the potbelly.

Rounded or full upper back. The neckline pulls down in back and up in front. If the garment was made with a center back seam, a dressmaker can let it out for you.

Bodywork

Clothes that used to look fabulous on us now look frumpy. Why? Our bodies change with age: weight shifts, shoulders slope, backs round, hips and thighs get fuller. Although we may still be the same size we were 10 years ago, we notice that our clothes have become too loose in some places and too tight in others.

To fit and flatter our new bodies, the styles we wear should change through the years. This isn't a matter of dressing our age—it's about dressing our *shape*.

Betzina offers suggestions for each age group in her home sewing pattern collection called "Today's Fit by Sandra Betzina." She developed the collection, which is based on extensive research of body shapes and measurements, in collaboration with Vogue Patterns.

Ages 24 to 34. This is the time to celebrate your youthful body. While a bit of padding may be creeping onto your hips, tummy, and thighs, there's no need to run for the cover of extra fabric. In fact, you can continue wearing fitted clothing.

But this is the time of life, cautions Betzina, when you have to acknowledge that your body is changing. If this means switching to a larger size for the lower half of the body, then so be it.

Ages 34 to 44. Your braless days are over, your waist is thickening, and a potbelly is starting to show.

Although you no longer have the body of a 20-year-old, you can continue wearing the same styles as a decade earlier by making a few concessions to your evolving shape. Experiment with wearing clothes that are looser in areas where you're not as full. A wrap top over a shaped skirt, for example, is figure-flattering yet still has enough room to skim fuller arms and other trouble spots.

A Point about Bra Fit

"A sagging bustline adds 10 pounds and 10 years to a woman's figure," writes image consultant Nancy Nix-Rice in her book *Looking Good: A Comprehensive Guide to Wardrobe Planning, Color, and Personal Style Development.*

To perk up your appearance, look for a bra that lifts the bust point to a more youthful location, midway between the base of the neck and the waist. Look for a bra that has built-in support: underwires, nonstretch straps, push-up pads, and other shapers.

Strap and band fit are equally important. The front and back elastic should wrap around the body in the same place, neither drooping nor pulling up in any spot, says Jan Larkey, an image consultant in Pittsburgh and author of *Flatter Your Figure.*

While on inspection, make sure that the elastic isn't stretched out. You should be able to slip a finger under the elastic. Now face front. If you have a bulge at each front arm crease (between the underarm and top of the shoulder) you need a larger cup.

First, measure around your rib cage directly beneath your bust and add 5 to the measurement. This is your bra size.

Then, measure the circumference around your full bust. The difference between the rib-cage and full-bust measurements indicates your cup size.

Difference	Cup Size
½ inch	AA
1 inch	A
2 inches	B
3 inches	C
4 inches	D
5 inches	DD or E
6 inches	DDD or F
7 inches	FF or G

Ages 44 to 54. Now your tummy measurement is beginning to exceed the circumference of your hips, so it's most important that garments drop straight from the fullest part of your lower body—usually the waist or high hips.

In pants, this translates into the classic trouser shape that Audrey Hepburn wore.

You can pull off a great suit look if the pants are topped with a longer jacket that has set-in sleeves (the top of the seam that joins the sleeve to the jacket is positioned at the upper arm/shoulder hinge).

Since there may be rolls between the bottom of the bra and the waist, garments that skim the body are

JEANS FOR COMFORT AND FIT

Many people feel that few things can give them a youthful look the way jeans can. The key is to find a style that tips its hat to the trends the kids are wearing without going overboard.

For example, when the twentysomething crowd is wearing an oversize and sloppy look, you can opt for a more relaxed fit and a low-rise waist that rests just below your belly button.

While it's easy to decide on a style that flatters your body, fit is harder to pin down. Some of us like jeans that are snug, while others prefer a looser feel.

"There really isn't a standard," explains Norma Willis, a design manager at the Lee Apparel Company in Merriam, Kansas. When a new style of jeans is in the development stage, however, a Lee fit model is asked to pull them on and move around: sit, bend to ensure that the upper legs aren't too tight, and walk a bit.

You can apply these same criteria the next time you shop for jeans. If the pants' rise is too short, the crotch will "cut" you when you sit.

As to choosing high-quality jeans, here are some tips.

Check seams. The best-made jeans have a lot of double-needle construction. Look for seams that have two lines of stitching, except along the outer leg/hip seamline. Here, single-seam construction does a better job over womanly curves.

Be a metal detector. A metal zipper is best because the chain teeth last longer.

Test bands. In a lightweight jean fabric, make sure that the waistband is stiffer so that it doesn't roll.

Look over hems. The best hem, featured on basic jeans, is rolled over double, which lasts longer than the wider, one-layer hem of fashion jeans.

Bring out the inner jean. At home with your new purchase, you can preserve the new color by washing the jeans inside out. Then let your pants drip-dry so that they don't shrink as much.

best. A center back seam is a plus because it can be let out to fit a rounded upper back and shoulders.

Ages 54 to 64. Your shoulders and back continue to round, a potbelly often becomes more pronounced, and your waist thickens.

Buy the best garments that you can afford. Generally, clothes that are more expensive are designed to fit the body better and have built-in structure and shape that camouflage problems. Opt for set-in sleeves and open necklines.

Consider a more relaxed look, suggests Betzina, by pushing or rolling up your sleeves. Avoid tuck-

ACCESSORIZE WITH STYLE

Classic or funky, your choice in accessories can define an outfit. A gold chain worn with a classic black dress is elegant. Now take off the necklace and put on an oversize watch to be instantly sporty.

These little touches—pins, necklaces, earrings, belts, and scarves—can make getting dressed so much fun. And once you have the basics, you can play with trends without taking a big bite out of your budget.

Bring a guide. Some image consultants advise you to shop alone so that you'll develop your own style. Princess Jenkins, image consultant and owner of Majestic Images International in New York City, suggests the opposite. Shop with youthful friends and family members. They know the trends, and they'll let you know when you've stepped over the line.

Think smaller. Image consultant Donna Fujii of San Francisco suggests borrowing a popular print, color, or motif that the twentysomething crowd is wearing in garments and buying yourself a belt or scarf with the same theme.

Out with the old. If you don't see young people wearing a particular kind of jewelry, then you shouldn't either, says Diana Kilgour, an image consultant in Vancouver, Canada. A lapel pin, for example, isn't popular now, so tuck your piece in a memory box rather than the jewelry box.

in looks because these emphasize a thick waist or tummy bulge.

Instead, consider an overshirt with narrow pants, or a T-shirt dress in a fabric that has drape without cling.

If you want to camouflage certain trouble spots, slip on a jacket with set-in sleeves.

The best way to determine what works for you is to experiment. In our teens, many of us spent hours trying on clothes. Soon, life got in the way, and there was little time to play with clothes.

It's time to start having fun again. "Don't get preconceived ideas of what looks good on you and what doesn't look good on you," says Betzina. "Try on different styles once a year, just like you did when you were young."

PART THREE

Youth
Makers

Attitude Is Everything

As a boy growing up in the eastern United States, John Deller, M.D., saw plenty of people around him retreat to their rocking chairs while they were still in their middle years. That's what you did after your working career was over—or so he thought. Then he moved out to the West Coast, where 80-year-olds play tennis and organize charity balls.

"Everybody in southern California thinks they're 25," says Dr. Deller, who's now an endocrinologist at the Heart Institute of the Desert in Rancho Mirage, California, and author of *Achieving Agelessness* and *The Palm Springs Formula for Healthy Living*.

Is there something in the water out there in sunny California? Have they found a secret supplement they are hiding from the rest of us? Maybe it's the laid-back lifestyle? According to Dr. Deller, the answer is much simpler: Aging is part biological, but also part psychological. How we *think* about aging determines how well we will actually do it. Our bodies' cells have a say in the matter, but for the most part, we control our relationship with Father Time because aging is mostly just a state of mind.

Acting Your Age

Just what is a youthful attitude? We all know what it isn't: It isn't behaving like a teenager—or even like a 20-year-old. It certainly doesn't mean trying to keep up with fashion fads of kids who are 20 years younger than you. You have worked too hard developing a sense of maturity over the years to fall into that trap.

A youthful state of mind combines a sense of self-esteem with a sense of all the possibilities life has to offer. It is knowing you can do whatever you put your mind to without a second thought about how many birthday candles you blew out at your last party. "The ones who work at the idea of keeping their options open, of pursuing all their interests, and of not looking at the calendar are the ones who achieve agelessness," Dr. Deller says.

It isn't easy. There's peer pressure to deal with.

You thought you left peer pressure behind in high school, right? Not so, unfortunately. Like acne, it's one of those things that happens to people of every age. It just gets more subtle as you get older.

People around you may have some pretty set-in-stone ideas about how you are supposed to behave at any given age, and without even realizing it, they may pressure you to slow down just when you feel like sprinting. Or you may apply the pressure yourself.

"You think because most people who are this age do or don't do this, you should, too. Being in a youthful state of mind means not giving too much of a damn what other people think. Don't be restricted by other people's stereotypes," says Albert Ellis, Ph.D., president of the Albert Ellis Institute for Rational Emotive Behavior Therapy in New York City and coauthor of *Optimal Aging* with Emmett Velten, Ph.D.

10 Attributes of a Youthful Mind

People in a perpetually youthful state of mind come from many different backgrounds, but they all possess personality traits that transcend age. Here are 10 qualities you'll find in youthful people, no matter what their chronological age.

Humor

"I was born in 1962. True. And the room next to me was 1963 . . ."—Joan Rivers. Age and getting older have always been the butt of jokes. Why? Because laughter puts things into perspective. If you can laugh at something, it can't be all that bad.

On the other hand, what kind of person comes to mind when you think of the word

---

SAY WHAT? WORDS THAT GIVE AWAY YOUR AGE

Maybe your appearance doesn't give away your age. And your attitude is more youthful than that of the kid who mows your lawn. So just what could tattle on you when it comes to how old you really are? Your mouth. Just one word or phrase from a bygone era can date you as fast as a paisley shirt and a pair of bell-bottoms. Here are a few to watch out for.

- Dungarees
- Bermuda (as in shorts)
- Nifty
- Icebox
- Brassiere
- Typewriter
- Record player
- Album
- Rouge
- Put on my face
- Hanky
- Lady-friend
- Jumping jacks
- Going steady
- When I was your age
- Gal or fella
- Calling everyone "Hon"
- Coed
- Hi-fi
- Far out
- Heavy
- Hip
- Necking
- Here comes the judge

Make up your own list. Your kids will be happy to point out new entries as they fall over laughing when you say them. In the meantime, "Peace and love!"

---

crotchety? You got it—humorless. Remember, a sense of humor got George Burns past 100. (Well, it certainly wasn't his cigar smoking that did it.) "Not only do older people who utilize humor seem younger in attitude, they actually look younger to me. On the other hand, when you see someone who is depressed and sullen, they look old and haggardly," says Steve Sultanoff, Ph.D., adjunct professor of psychology at Pepperdine University in Malibu, California, and president of the American Association for Therapeutic Humor.

No need to take pratfalls on banana peels.

WOMEN ASK WHY

Why does time seem to go by faster the older I get?

Perhaps no one told you just how busy the middle years would be. You are potentially at the peak of your career, your children and your parents rely on you, and you are trying to fit a social life and extracurricular activities in as well. So you have a lot to do and not enough time in which to do it.

That sense of being rushed creates a feeling that time is fleeting and that life is moving at a rapid pace. And that's the way your brain actually registers it. Why? Handling too many tasks at once interferes with the brain's ability to accurately measure time. When you think back years ago, it is not that time went slower, you just had a lot less to do.

The natural process of aging may also alter your sense of time passing. Each of us has what experts call an internal clock. This clock enables you to reasonably measure time in your head. Therefore, your perception of time relies heavily on two processes in the brain: memory and attention, both of which slow down a bit as you get older, throwing your perception of time off track.

This natural slowdown combined with managing a hectic schedule and numerous responsibilities knocks your internal clock a bit off center. Your brain handles all these factors in a way that makes you feel like time whizzes by faster than before.

Expert consulted
Deborah Harrington, Ph.D.
Research scientist
Veteran Affairs Medical Center
Albuquerque, New Mexico

tain comedian, slapstick humor, or funny props? Some people never take the time to seek out different brands of humor and just assume they are laughing-impaired.

Surround yourself with laughter. Once you have identified what humor you like, keep it around. Buy movies and books by your favorite comedians and pull them out when you need to laugh. Tack hilarious cartoons or quotes around your home or office. Carry clown noses or silly props with you and yank them out. "I carry Groucho glasses and clown noses everywhere I go," Dr. Sultanoff proudly admits. This is not a requirement, however.

Look for humor in serious situations. Your teenager has just come home an hour past curfew. You mete out a punishment. You're angry; she's resentful. And that adolescent attitude is just about to send you up the wall when . . . a fly lands on her nose, she crosses her eyes, and she smacks herself trying to get it.

Dr. Sultanoff says that a good laugh could be what you need during a tense moment to bring in a new perspective.

Hang out with children. Children, in their innocence, are inherently funny. Spend some time with children and learn to laugh and play like them, Dr. Sultanoff says. If children aren't in your circle of friends, just hang out with funny people or even furry friends that make you laugh.

Give yourself permission. Afraid people will laugh at you? Well, that's the point, Dr. Sul-

There are simpler ways to get the humor rolling. Here are just a few.

Find humor you enjoy. Does Robin Williams make you laugh or make you sick? Identify what types of humor you like, Dr. Sultanoff says. Do you enjoy jokes, cartoons, a certanoff says. In order to delight in humor, you must allow yourself to be funny. Some people get so wrapped up in the seriousness of life that they won't permit themselves the enjoyment of humor. Give yourself the green light, and you will feel lighthearted and younger, he says.

Optimism

Just think about what it means to be a pessimist: You believe that bad events are all your fault, that misfortune will follow you always, and that life will consistently turn out for the worst. No wonder it ages you.

Martin E. P. Seligman, Ph.D., a leading expert on optimism and author of *Learned Optimism*, says in his book that optimists age better, live longer, catch fewer infectious diseases, and have stronger immune systems than pessimists. Studies have also shown that pessimists give up more easily and get depressed more often. An optimist has a firm grip on reality but also recognizes that just about any event—good or bad—has advantages. Here's how to look on the bright side of anything.

Argue with yourself. According to Dr. Seligman's groundbreaking book, dispute your pessimistic beliefs. For example, let's say that you hand in a report and the boss doesn't like it. Your first reaction is that you will be fired. But cross-examine your thought processes. Will you really be fired for one not-so-hot report after years of good work? Can't you go back and make the revisions she wants? Often, you'll realize that you blow negative events out of proportion.

Turn bad events into good motivators. An optimist views a negative event as an opportunity, Dr. Ellis says. If you don't like your job and think you will be miserable forever, use that as a catalyst to find a new job. If you are sad because family or friends moved away, use your newfound free time to find new interests or meet new people.

Seek out the silver lining. Perhaps you just got a new job. A few weeks after you start, your car breaks down, your dishwasher blows up, and your roof needs repairs. Now you can think: What terrible luck I have. I've just started earning a decent paycheck, and all my money's gone out the window. Or you can think: These things were going to happen eventually, so it's really lucky that they happened now that I have a new job, when I can afford the repairs. A simple change in perspective can make your life a lot more enjoyable, Dr. Ellis says.

Curiosity

Spend any amount of time with a 4-year-old, and the word you're likely to hear most often is *why*. Spend the same amount of time with a 44-year-old, and *why* may be the word you hear least. "If you look at children, they are curious about the world. Unfortunately, we lose that as we get older," says William Strawbridge, Ph.D., an epidemiologist at the Public Health Institute in Berkeley, California.

Why? Perhaps we felt foolish too many times for asking "silly" questions, or maybe we just stopped caring about the hows and whys of life and began taking it at face value.

To recapture that sense of wonder and inquisitiveness is to recapture part of your youth, Dr. Strawbridge says. As a bonus, curiosity leads you to other interests in life such as new hobbies, new experiences, and possibly even new careers. Want to know how you can recapture that precious part of yourself?

Ask why. It is such a simple question, but one that people often don't ask, Dr. Strawbridge says. Start to ask yourself and others why. Why is the sky blue? Why do I want this job? Why can't I take up a new hobby?

Don't accept "just because." It's easy to take someone else's word for something, but you will miss out on the excitement of your own discoveries. It's better to do your own homework, Dr. Strawbridge says. Ask if there is a better way of doing things at home, at work, or even at play. Albert Einstein based his success on simple curiosity: "The important thing is not to stop questioning."

Dig into things. If something intrigues you, look into it, Dr. Strawbridge says. Want to know how a computer works? Tinker with one. Then read books and newspapers and get on the Internet to learn more about the subject. You can take the same approach with any interest from sewing to botany. Get hands-on experience and immerse yourself in some research at the same time.

Adventure

In 1998, Sister Clarice Lolich celebrated her 80th birthday by skydiving out of an airplane. Not that this type of adventure was new for this nun and former aerospace education specialist with NASA: She has also bungee-jumped, parasailed, and whitewater-rafted.

She never lost her sense of adventure, an important key to staying young, says Dr. Ellis. Emotionally healthy people take risks. But as some people get older, they become more cautious. By regaining that sense of adventure, you are very likely to feel younger and more alive, he adds.

You don't have to jump out of an airplane or take a trip to the Amazon to partake of an adventure (unless you want to, of course). A trip to a new restaurant, a new job, or a new vacation can fill that bill very well. "You can take many risks, both large and small," Dr. Ellis says. Here are some places to start.

MAKING THE MOST OF MIDLIFE CRISIS

The term *midlife crisis* comes to us from art history. In studying the careers of some of the world's most famous artists, one author noticed that they all had shown a dramatic change in their work after age 35. They seemed far more concerned with images that reflected their own sense of mortality than with pictures that celebrated the past.

You know you've hit a midlife crisis when you start to reevaluate just about everything around you—your job, your relationships, your achievements. "You no longer feel secure with the status quo, but you aren't exactly sure how to proceed. What you are sure of is that life doesn't last forever and that you need to make some decisions about how you will proceed with the rest of yours," says Leonard Felder, Ph.D., a psychologist in Los Angeles and author of *The 10 Challenges*.

Many people reach this midlife point and reflect on the mistakes they have made over the years. Instead, they should be contemplating their futures. "Most women that I see go back and beat themselves up for some decision they made years ago and think that will help them get through a midlife crisis. It is not about finding a guilty party. It is about making excellent choices," says Dr. Felder.

Eat exotically. Take your tastebuds on a trip to another country by dining at an ethnic restaurant, Dr. Ellis says. Eating new foods can be an exciting escapade.

Change your travel plans. Do you go to the same vacation spot year in and year out? Pick a different destination, Dr. Ellis says. You don't need to travel to Bali or Australia. Simply navigating your way in a new city or locale can bring out the adventurer in you.

Introduce yourself. Meeting people often turns into an adventure, Dr. Ellis says. Introduce yourself to new people at work or join a special-interest group or social club. Unless you

What triggers a midlife crisis? It can be the illness or death of someone your own age, watching younger people climb past you on the ladder to professional or personal success, or simply feeling that there has to be something more to get you out of bed each morning. Each of these events provides the perfect opportunity to make positive changes. Here's how Dr. Felder says you can make the most of a midlife crisis.

❥ Make small changes first. "People often bolt from a job or a relationship that wasn't really so bad. Then they regret leaving when it is all over," he says. Identify what you don't enjoy about your job, your relationships. Then change that aspect of your life. Small changes make a world of difference.

❥ Seek fulfillment elsewhere. Perhaps your job and relationships are healthy, but you feel that you're still missing something. Take classes in subjects that interest you, volunteer, get active in your community. "Find those activities and values you've put on hold," he says. Many times those deepening activities offer the fulfillment you've been looking for.

❥ Look way into the future. Maybe it is unrealistic for you to quit your 9-to-5 job and become a gourmet chef right now. But who is to say you can't do that when you retire? Use your midlife crisis to figure out what your dreams are, then start laying the groundwork now for your later years.

being to a number of traits you develop as you mature: experience, a better attitude toward life, a greater sense of living in the moment. "As you get older, you know yourself better. You know what makes you happy. And you are better able to do these things that make you happy," he says. So in order to be happy and youthful, embrace your maturity—don't hide it. "A lot of women try to act young. Why deny that valuable experience, knowledge, and know-how?" he says.

Share your life experience. Share your knowledge and wisdom with friends, family, and coworkers. If you know how to do something better, speak up.

Value what you have done. Think about all you have already accomplished in your life, he says. Enjoy those achievements instead of thinking about what you could have, should have, or would have done—or what you still have to do. You still look toward the future, of course, but don't forget to cherish your past as well.

Savor the moment. In studying age and happiness, Dr. Mroczek found that older people report a greater sense of well-being because they enjoy the moment at hand and worry less about the future. "They stop and smell the roses. They look at sunsets, enjoy the blue sky. They are less future-oriented," he says. Enjoy each day and what it brings, he advises. Good advice at any age.

live on a desert island, new people are everywhere you look.

Maturity

It's a scientific fact: The older you are, the happier you are. A study of 2,700 people from ages 25 to 75 conducted at Fordham University in New York City found that happiness increases with age. "The typical stereotype of the older, depressed individual is just that—a stereotype," says Daniel K. Mroczek, Ph.D., assistant professor of psychology at Fordham University and study author.

Dr. Mroczek attributes this increase in well-

Knowledge

Henry Ford perfectly captured the secret of staying young when he said, "Anyone who stops learning is old, whether at 20 or 80. Anyone who keeps learning stays young. The greatest thing in life is to keep your mind young."

Research has discovered the role for learning in healthy aging. A study at the Public Health Institute found that people with 12 years or more of education were healthier in their later years than those who had less schooling. But the study's author, Dr. Strawbridge, takes his results beyond classroom experience. Building knowledge is a lifelong endeavor. "Learning follows you all your life. If you are 45, you are not going back to high school. But you can certainly do things to learn and improve your mental activity," he says. Here's how to increase your knowledge as long as you live.

Get back to class. There is a plethora of ways to go back to school now: community colleges, adult education centers, night learning classes, summer programs for adults, Dr. Strawbridge says. And now, unlike in high school, you can take whatever courses you want.

Read, read, read. Being a voracious reader makes you a voracious learner. Beyond books, newspapers, and magazines, the Internet opens up a whole new world of knowledge, Dr. Ellis says.

Use the tube. The television set doesn't always have to numb your mind. Used the right way, this medium is a form of education. Instructional videos can lead to new hobbies or activities. Educational programming such as that on PBS can teach you about science, nature, history, and the arts.

Enthusiasm

A reporter once asked fashion designer Gabrielle "Coco" Chanel about her age during an interview. Chanel, then 86, replied, "I will tell you that my age varies according to the day and the people I happen to be with. When I'm bored, I feel very old, and since I'm extremely bored with you, I'm going to be one

thousand years old if you don't get out of here at once."

Boredom—and surrounding yourself with boring people—can age you instantly. Having an enthusiastic outlook on life means being interested in life, in hobbies, in having fun, and in other people. According to Dr. Ellis, most people are healthier and happier when vitally absorbed in something other than themselves. To grow younger as you age, you need a creative interest as well as daily meaningful interaction with others.

Discover or revisit hobbies. Midlife is a great time to find new interests and hobbies. Rediscover creative activities that you loved to do in the past but lost touch with over the years because of a lack of time, Dr. Ellis says. Even something as simple as a hobby gives you a reason to be enthusiastic about life, and that keeps you ageless.

"It has to be something that is genuine, that you want to do. It can't be 'Now I should basket-weave.' You need to really feel charged up about this," Dr. Deller adds.

Keep up with friends and family. As life moves on, sometimes you lose touch with friends and family, or you don't make many new friends. But you want to work on those ties that bind.

According to a study of 65- to 95-year-old people by Dr. Strawbridge, those who had five or more people with whom they had close contact were twice as likely to "age successfully," meaning that they lead healthy and active lives well into older age. These close relationships build an instant support system and naturally keep you active and enthusiastic about a world other than your own.

Spend time with friends and family of all ages, Dr. Deller suggests, to keep in touch with all aspects of life.

Get involved in your community. Becoming active in your community kills two birds with one stone: It gives you an interest and provides a way to meet people, Dr. Ellis says. Join local organizations and school boards or attend government meetings.

Compassion

Empathy and understanding may be hard traits to develop, but they often reap benefits for both the giver and receiver. To be able to care, offer help, and show concern for others generates a joy that subtracts years off your age. "You do it because you get joy in doing it. I think that is really quite a healthy attitude," Dr. Sultanoff says.

Being compassionate doesn't mean that you compromise your ideals. "You don't have to accept what they do, but you accept them. When you do that, you actually enjoy helping others instead of criticizing others," Dr. Ellis says. You also fulfill the most basic human desire: to feel wanted and needed.

Become a volunteer. Find a cause you believe in and donate your time and energy, Dr. Strawbridge says. Studies show that volunteering benefits both your body and mind. A national survey of 3,330 volunteers found that they experienced a "helper's high," a sense of euphoria after helping others. They also reported an increased sense of self-worth and better perceived health, which is a predictor of future health and longevity.

Donate your skills. Maybe volunteering for an organization isn't your style, so contribute what you do best. "If you are an accountant,

WOMAN TO WOMAN

She Never Says No to a New Experience

Sylvia Palkowski, 62, a retired secretary from Fort Walton Beach, Florida, is always surprised to see an older woman looking back at her in the mirror—because she doesn't feel any older than 40. She finds all sorts of ways to retain her youth, from doing crafts to tap dancing. Here, she tells how fulfilling a lifelong dream made her feel like a kid again.

I think you're never too old to dream. And we all have dreams we haven't realized. I always wanted to be in a beauty pageant as a young girl but never really had the chance. Then about 10 years ago, I heard about the Miss Senior Okaloosa County Pageant here in Florida.

Being in the pageant turned out to be all I had imagined it would be—and more. Everything leading up to it was so much fun: meeting the seven other contestants, being interviewed by the judges, and walking through the dress rehearsal.

The night of the pageant, we all gathered backstage to primp and prettify before it was our turn to go out on the stage. I felt all aflutter like I was 18 again.

When it was my turn, I went in front of the microphone and summed up my philosophy of life, which I based largely on a prayer by St. Francis of Assisi. For the talent portion, I performed a comedy takeoff of an Erma Bombeck routine. Then it was time for the evening gown competition. We paraded onstage decked out in our most elegant attire. I wore an exquisite turquoise dress with a full skirt and beaded jacket.

The most memorable part of the pageant for me was what went on backstage. The camaraderie. Everybody helping everybody else with that zipper that wouldn't zip or that seam that came undone. Comforting the woman who goofed and encouraging the one about to go on.

I wasn't crowned the winner, but I didn't care a whit about winning. I did it just to do it. To be a part of it. To see what it's like. And it was just wonderful. I made lots of memories—and friends. And when I found out that one of the contestants was 90 years old, I felt like a spring chicken. No matter what our ages, we all made our childhood dreams come true. No one should ever give up a dream. Not ever.

help people with their taxes. Use your skills to help others. It doesn't have to be heavy involvement," Dr. Strawbridge says.

Get a pet. People aren't the only creatures that deserve love and affection; furry and feathered ones do, too. A pet large or small brings out the kindness in you. "You care for another being that totally relies on you," says Dr. Sultanoff.

Open-Mindedness

Nothing can make you feel older than being stuck in a rut. Same cereal for breakfast, same route to work, same vacation every year, same laundry day. Although this monotonous routine sounds terrible, some balk when faced with doing something different. The rut may be boring, but it is safe and comfortable.

If you want to maintain a youthful outlook on life, Dr. Ellis says that you need to be open-minded. "Healthy and mature people tend to be flexible in their thinking, open to change, and accepting in their views of people. They do not make rigid rules for themselves or others," he says.

Change your daily routine. Little changes spice up a routine and slowly get you used to trying something different. Take a different route to work. If you usually brush your teeth then brush your hair, switch. Try a new shade of eye shadow or lipstick. "Do things that aren't very important to you, but that at least break the mold of your everyday life," Dr. Sultanoff says.

Look for alternatives. There is always another way of doing things, another point of view. Don't discount them, Dr. Ellis says. In fact, seek them out. "People think they must do X and Y,

and they don't realize there are always alternatives that are often better," he adds.

Don't make absolutes. Perhaps you always go to your sister's house for Thanksgiving. But you can't stand her husband, other family members nag you to death, and you'd rather be anywhere else. Then why not be anywhere else? Dr. Ellis asks. There is no law that says you have to do something. "You have flexibility and the power to choose," he says.

Faith

Even science has gotten into the act of faith. Experts from Georgetown University School of Medicine in Washington, D.C., and Duke University Medical Center in Durham, North Carolina, who were reviewing studies on religion and health found that religious commitment may prevent many medical problems such as illness, depression, substance abuse, and even early death.

In many cases, faith provides a sense of being cared for, loved, and valued—all feelings that enhance your well-being and feed your youthful outlook. Spirituality also embraces the wisdom that comes with age. "Religion helps you to understand that growing old is not a bad thing," Dr. Strawbridge says.

Get involved. If you are a member of a faith or interested in becoming one, get involved in a church or temple. You become more active in the faith itself, and it often leads to social activities and volunteer work, Dr. Strawbridge says.

Find your own spirituality. Organized religion is not the only avenue to faith. Find your own way to celebrate your beliefs, Dr. Strawbridge says. Perhaps sitting quietly in a natural setting gets you in touch with your spiritual side.

Getting Your Weight Right

You gain a lot as you reach your middle years: understanding, control, self-confidence, wisdom, stature, freedom—and, unfortunately, weight. Whether it's a joke of Mother Nature's or an accident of evolution, a woman's scale and her age creep up together as she reaches her thirties, forties, and beyond.

All sorts of factors fight against you in your battle with extra pounds during this time of your life. "It's not hard to gain weight. There are all kinds of metabolic changes that promote weight gain as you get older," says Susan Roberts, Ph.D., professor of nutrition and psychiatry and chief of the energy metabolism laboratory at Tufts University in Boston.

First off, your body's metabolism slows down. In other words, you burn fewer calories during an activity now than you would have 20 years ago. "Even athletes have decreased energy expenditure with aging," Dr. Roberts says.

You also tend to be less physically active at this stage of your life than when you were younger, which slows the calorie burn even more. And to top it all off, muscle mass naturally decreases with age. Since muscle uses up more

energy fuel than any other kind of tissue, including fat, having less muscle diminishes your calorie burn still further.

It sounds as if we're doomed, but there's reason to take heart. We aren't supposed to look like we did when we were 25, and a little extra weight may not hurt us, especially if we are physically active. On average, women gain 10 to 15 pounds by age 60, says Michael Hamilton, M.D., program and medical director of the Diet Fitness Center at Duke University in Durham, North Carolina.

The key during these years is to find a *healthy* weight. Here's how to find what's the right weight for you and what you need to do to keep it there.

Weighing In

Ahh, the dreaded scale. Women have learned to treat its revolving numbers as the measure of truth when it comes to their worth and health. They look for that one magic number that will tell them everything is all right. But science has moved beyond the actual digits that show up on the scale and has found that factors other than weight alone have much more significant influence on your health.

Many weight experts now rely on the body mass index, better known as the BMI, to gauge your well-being. The BMI compares your height to your weight. A healthy BMI usually falls into the 20 to 25 range, says Susan Fried, Ph.D., associate professor of nutritional sciences at Rutgers University in New Brunswick, New Jersey. So if you had a BMI of 21 when you were in your twenties but now have a BMI of 23, you are still considered to be at a normal, healthy weight.

If you're in the over-25 range, it may be time to make some changes. A BMI of 25 to 30 is considered overweight; and a BMI over 30 is in the obese category. If you find yourself in either of those ranges, you'd do your health a favor by losing some weight. Why? Because numbers above 25 have been linked to increased rates of heart disease, diabetes, and breast cancer. Numbers above 30 have been even more closely linked with these problems.

Here's how to determine your BMI: Multiply your weight in pounds by 705. Divide the result by your height in inches, then divide that result by your height in inches again. So if you are 145 pounds and 66 inches tall, your BMI would be 23.4, well within the healthy range.

But BMI isn't the whole story. Where you add on weight may be as important as how much, says Dr. Fried. Women who carry extra fat in their abdomens are at greater risk for weight-related diseases than are those who gain in their thighs, hips, or butts. So researchers

REAL-LIFE SCENARIO
Why Is She So Thin and Old-Looking?

Marie is 39 years old, although from the look of her, you'd guess she was closer to 59, which someone recently did say. She was crushed. She had thought she looked great because she had never allowed herself to put on an ounce since she'd gotten out of college, as so many other women her age had. Then, after the birth of her last daughter, she'd gotten back down to within 7 pounds of her normal weight, when she plateaued. She was horrified. To her, fat meant unattractive. She immediately cut her food intake down to 1,000 calories a day. She's never been so thin—right down to the hollows in her cheeks, her sunken eyes, and her frail-looking shoulders. And lately her back and knees have been hurting her, and more often than not, she has a cold. She thought she'd chosen a healthy way to live. What's gone wrong?

Marie has two serious misconceptions about her weight. Her first is equating low weight— even lower-than-normal—with attractiveness and good health. Her second is allowing her weight to control her self-esteem. Both beliefs are making her look and feel old before her time.

The key to reaching and maintaining a healthy weight is to do the all right things *within reason*. If Marie ate a balanced diet and exercised regularly, her weight would fall to where

have devised another guideline to assess weight and health risk: your waist circumference. If your waist is larger than 35 inches, says Dr. Fried, you may be at higher risk for heart disease, stroke, diabetes, high blood pressure, and certain cancers.

The BMI and waist circumference act as good general guidelines, but it is possible to be perfectly fit with a BMI over 25. And you can be out of shape and live a nonhealthy lifestyle and have a BMI under 25. Here are some other criteria to help you decide where your weight should be.

her body needed it to be. When Marie was 7 pounds over her pre-pregnancy weight, she was at no higher risk for health problems than she had been before getting pregnant. But now that she has reached what she considers a "healthy" weight, she's experiencing all kinds of symptoms, and she looks unhealthy.

Why? Her body is telling her that it doesn't want to be that thin. If she insists on remaining at that weight, she'll have to live like a Spartan for the rest of her life. No person could keep up such a lifestyle.

Marie must also begin to recognize that a number on a scale does not define her worth as a person. Right now, her identification with what she weighs has turned into an unhealthy obsession. There's a very good chance that, no matter how many pounds she loses, she'll never be satisfied. And as long as she links her body weight with her self-esteem, she'll never feel good about herself.

If Marie wants to move beyond the scale and live life completely, she'll have to start defining herself in different ways—by her value as a mother, a friend, a wife, a worker.

Expert consulted
Gary Foster, Ph.D.
Clinical director of the weight and eating disorders program
University of Pennsylvania School of Medicine
Philadelphia

Fitness level. If you carry an extra 10 to 15 pounds but are physically active and can do daily tasks—walk up and down hills, climb steps, run to catch a bus—without a problem, then you are probably fine, says Jill Kanaley, Ph.D., assistant professor of exercise science and director of the human performance laboratory at Syracuse University in New York. If you aren't fit and you have a problem getting around, then your weight may pose a health risk.

Family history. If your parents are overweight and have problems such as high blood pressure, high cholesterol, or diabetes, chances are the extra weight may cause the same problems for you, says Dr. Kanaley. But if Mom and Dad were overweight all their lives, yet were fit and lived into their eighties or nineties, you have less to worry about.

Other risk factors. Women who are carrying a few extra pounds but are otherwise healthy shouldn't worry too much. "They shouldn't beat themselves up over their weight," Dr. Kanaley says. But if you have high cholesterol, high blood pressure, or diabetes, losing the extra weight could lessen your risk of developing serious health problems in the future.

If you do need to lose weight, you don't necessarily have to go from a BMI of 30 to the low 20s to get health benefits. Expert panels and government guidelines have determined that a 5- to 10-percent drop in body weight—maintained for one year—should be considered a success, says Gary Foster, Ph.D., clinical director of the weight and eating disorders program at the University of Pennsylvania School of Medicine in Philadelphia. In other words, if you weigh 200 pounds and are considered overweight, a loss of 20 pounds would be a reasonable and healthy goal. Why 10 percent? It is a realistic goal, it is easier to maintain, and various studies have shown that just a 10-percent loss improves many of the medical conditions associated with excess weight such as diabetes and high blood pressure, Dr. Foster says.

Say Goodbye to Dieting

There's a reason trendy diets go out of style as fast as go-go boots and beehive hairdos: They don't work. As you talk to weight-loss experts, you'll hear over and over again that there is no magic weight-loss diet. If you drastically cut back on calories to lose weight, the pounds will come flocking back once you start to eat normally again.

The not-so-secret secret to weight loss and control is not an eating plan with a sexy name and lots of hype, but a healthy, low-fat diet that emphasizes fruits, grains, and vegetables. If you make it part of your lifestyle, you won't have to worry about gaining pounds back. "Fad diets come and go. Over and over we see that the only thing that really works is a balanced, healthy diet with moderation," says Lorna Pascal, R.D., nutrition coordinator at the Dave Winfield Nutrition Center at the Hackensack University Medical Center in Hackensack, New Jersey.

When it comes to planning and eating meals, remember these tips to help keep the pounds off.

Fill up with fiber. Not only is fiber good for you, but it fills you up more quickly and with fewer calories, which prevents you from eating more. A study at the Brooke Army Medical Center at Fort Sam Houston, Texas, found that pectin, a soluble fiber found in the skins of fruits and vegetables, made people feel fuller longer. To get more fiber, base your meals on fruits, vegetables, legumes, and whole grains, such as whole-wheat bread, brown rice, and whole-grain breakfast cereals, says Melanie Polk, R.D., director of nutrition education at the American Institute for Cancer Research in Washington, D.C.

Get low-fat and lean. Each gram of fat contains more calories than a gram of protein or carbohydrate. Eating a high-fiber diet full of

---

WOMAN TO WOMAN

Her Self-Image Improved after She Took an Honest Look at Herself

Ever since she had to buy a dress at the "chubette" department when she was a preteen, Mary Talbot, a 35-year-old marketing/public relations executive from Barrington, Rhode Island, has waged a war with her weight. For most of her adolescence and adult life, she practically starved herself and worked her body to the max, all to keep herself in a size 12 dress. Then a trip to the doctor's office made her realize that her obsession with weight was controlling her life and ruining her self-esteem. This is her story.

For most of my twenties, I stayed around a size 12. People who looked at me would say that I was average, maybe a bit chubby, but never heavy or overweight. They didn't know that I was working out five days a week and hardly eating. I ran at least 25 miles a week. My typical diet was a big salad, one yogurt, maybe a bagel, and some type of protein for dinner. And that was it. I figure I ate only 1,000 to 1,250 calories a day. Despite this, I was never thinner than "normal."

The constant obsessing about my weight and lack of self-esteem affected my relationships. In social settings, I was withdrawn. I also tended to let all the wrong men into my life. That's because I knew the good men out there weren't

---

fruits, vegetables, and whole grains naturally helps you cut down on fat, Polk says. Also, limit your use of oils and butter and switch to dairy products like fat-free milk, low-fat cheese, and low-fat yogurt. If you eat meat, choose moderate portions of skinless chicken and turkey and lean cuts of red meat, such as top round, bottom round, and top sirloin.

Be moderate. No food is bad if you don't eat too much of it. "We live in a super-sized world," Pascal says. Even people who choose low-fat fare will gain weight if they eat too much. You can enjoy just about any food as long as you enjoy it in moderation.

really attracted to women who have low self-esteem. So when an attractive man did approach, I was skeptical of his motives.

On top of all that, I was terribly frustrated that I couldn't get the scale to move. In fact, I got to a point where I felt so frustrated that I went to my doctor and told him, "Here is what I have eaten for the last 7 days." I tracked every morsel I put into my mouth, and it was my typical diet. What was wrong with me? And he said that I was basically starving myself and had been for years—that I actually wasn't eating enough. He told me my blood pressure was low, my cholesterol was low, and that I was extremely fit. He said, "Maybe you weren't meant to be a thin person."

After that, I decided that I was going to have to be satisfied with myself or I was going to waste all this energy on excessive dieting and exercise. Life is too short for that. I still lead a very active and healthy lifestyle: I swim three or four nights a week, I weight train and I eat right, but I don't worry about the number on the scale.

I am happier and I feel younger now than I did 5 years ago because I am not obsessed about my weight. I wish I had had this kind of self-confidence 5, 10, 15 years ago. It feels great walking down the beach in my bathing suit. I am who I am, and I am proud of it.

Eat with all your senses. It's easy to gulp down a meal without enjoying it, then end up still feeling unsatisfied. If you focus more on your food, a little will go a long way, Polk says. Look at the plate and study the colors and textures. "Get the visual enjoyment," she adds. Then close your eyes and smell the aroma of the meal. As you put a small bite into your mouth, pay attention to the texture and taste of each and every morsel. Slowly chew and savor the food before swallowing, she says. "You'll satisfy all your senses and realize that you don't need to eat as much food to get the enjoyment out of it."

Size up serving sizes. When is a bagel not a bagel? When it's really four bagels. Just because you eat one of something doesn't mean it's a single serving. Many foods—such as a big bagel—are actually four servings of bread. When you're eating foods that come in bulk, such as rice or pastas, read their labels and figure out exactly what a serving size is, Pascal says. Measure out how much food you eat and compare it to the label to see how many calories and grams of fat you are actually getting. Once you learn servings, you'll be able to judge with your eye how much you should eat.

Ask for a doggie bag first. Because they're so busy, many women find themselves eating out a lot these days. Restaurant serving sizes can be up to four times what a regular serving size should be. To make sure that you don't overdo it, ask for the doggie bag first, Polk says. Put half of the meal away before you even start to eat.

Make veggies the centerpiece. In a typical American meal, meat is often the star. Vegetables and whole grains just garnish the main event. Break out of that mindset, Polk says. Make vegetables and whole grains the centerpiece. If you do have meat, make it a small side dish.

Utilize spices and flavors. Fat isn't the only way to flavor food. Polk suggests using nonfat sauces such as teriyaki, flavored vinegars, or no-fat salad dressing. Season vegetables and meats with herbs and spices to add flavor without fat.

Be prepared. If you don't have any healthy low-fat food around, it's easy to fall into a fat-eating trap. Stock up your pantry with a few items to make sure that you can always fix a quick-and-easy, tasty meal: brown rice, whole-grain spaghetti, beans, salsa, frozen vegetables, canned fruit, low-fat pasta sauce, and low-fat chicken broth. Polk points out that many combinations of these items can make a quick, tasty meal.

Snack on fruits and vegetables. Snacking isn't evil when you're trying to lose or maintain weight—as long as you pick healthy, low-fat snacks, Polk says. When you feel the hunger set in before meals, try fresh or canned fruit, whole-wheat crackers, vegetables such as baby carrots, or a glass of low-fat or fat-free milk.

Putting Exercise into Everyday Events

Exercise is important at every stage of life. It makes you stronger and helps battle high blood pressure, heart disease, and osteoporosis. But as you get older, exercise takes on a much more important role in your weight-loss/weight-control regimen.

Exercise not only helps you lose weight but also helps you keep it off. Studies have shown that women who continue to exercise regularly are more successful at maintaining weight loss than those who do not, Dr. Foster says.

Aerobic exercise also gets rid of abdominal fat, which causes more health problems than extra pounds on any other part of the body, Dr. Fried says.

Experts now say that making movement part of your everyday life is just as effective as going to a gym a couple of times a week, Dr. Fried says.

"A lot of people think, 'If I am not out there running 5 miles a day, I am not exercising.' Now we are recommending 15 to 20 minutes of some activity—no matter how simple—every day," Dr. Kanaley adds. A study at the Cooper Institute for Aerobics Research in Dallas revealed that lifestyle physical activity—like taking a brisk walk or raking leaves—was as effective as a structured exercise program in improving physical activity, heart and respiratory fitness, blood pressure, and body fat on healthy but sedentary adults.

Whether you already have an exercise program or you're just starting out, read the following to learn how easy it is to mix physical activity into everyday tasks.

Walk this way. Exercise trends may come and go (remember Jazzercise?), but walking is still the cheapest and easiest exercise you can do. A ½-hour walk a day is a good way to start. If you can't do it in one chunk, take several shorter walks throughout the day. If you can, make walking your primary mode of transportation, Dr. Fried says. If you can walk to the store instead of driving, do so.

Count your steps. According to Dr. Hamilton, you should take at least 10,000 steps a day. Instead of boggling your mind counting each step in your head, you can track your daily physical activity with a pedometer. Dr. Hamilton wears his, which cost him about $24, on his belt or underwear. It measures every step you take so that you can make sure you reach your 10,000 steps a day, he says. If Dr. Hamilton comes up short some days, he knows he needs to take a walk or make it up the next day. "I had to drive someplace one day, so I only made 6,000 steps. But the next day, I took a 2-mile walk and registered 13,000," he says.

Get down in the dirt. Whether you get dirty in your garden or clean your house, both activities burn off calories. "Spending a day in your garden is a great workout," Dr. Kanaley says. And although cleaning may not sound like fun, think of it as a weight-loss exercise instead of housework.

Become a fidget. Don't think that finger tapping and stretching at your desk help you lose weight? Guess again. Researchers at the Mayo Clinic in Rochester, Minnesota, fed an extra 1,000 calories a day to 16 volunteers for 8 weeks. The volunteers also wore instruments that measured their energy output. The study found that those who fidgeted stayed slim. Small movements such as finger and toe tapping, maintaining good posture, stretching, and standing up often burned calories that would have been stored as fat. You too can become a fidget. Get up and walk around every 15 minutes or so, stretch, and just keep moving during the day.

Count the little things. By taking an extra few steps, you burn off a few more calories

---

THE PRICE OF PREGNANCY

After gaining anywhere from 20 to 50 pounds per child, you'd think that pregnancy would contribute to the weight problem of many women. Not so, at least for a majority of moms. Two studies have discovered that most women either go back to their pre-pregnancy weight or just a few pounds above it.

A study at the Karolinska Hospital in Stockholm, Sweden, followed 1,423 pregnant women until a year after their deliveries. On average, the women were about a pound heavier than they were before their pregnancies. Thirty percent actually dropped below their pre-pregnancy weight, while 56 percent gained anywhere between zero and 11 pounds. Only 14 percent kept more than 11 pounds. Another study at the University of Iceland looked at 200 women 2 years after giving birth. About 89 percent of the women got back to their pre-pregnancy weight.

Studies haven't shown any metabolic process that would keep weight on after a pregnancy, says Jill Kanaley, Ph.D., assistant professor of exercise science and director of the human performance laboratory at Syracuse University in New York. Whether a woman gains or loses weight after a pregnancy depends on how much she eats and exercises.

---

and get a little more exercise into your day. "Be as inefficient as possible," Dr. Hamilton says. He suggests some simple yet worthwhile things to do.

- Park your car a few blocks away and walk.
- Avoid revolving doors. Open the door yourself.
- Carry your own bags. Never use the wheels on luggage.
- Use the stairs whenever possible.
- Make several trips when taking out the trash, carrying in the dishes, doing the laundry.
- Make the most of litter. When you see it, squat down, pick it up, and throw it away.

Lifting the Pounds

Getting rid of the pounds isn't always the best way to fit into a smaller dress size. In many cases, adding weight—as in free weights—is the perfect way to slim down. "Resistance training deserves its place in the components of fitness for women," says Harvey Newton, a certified strength and conditioning specialist and executive director of the National Strength and Conditioning Association (NSCA) in Colorado Springs, Colorado.

Even if you don't lose a single pound on the scale, weight training tones and firms up the body you have, making it appear sleeker and slimmer. After all, a toned 145-pound body looks much better than a nontoned 145-pound body, Newton says. And it can add a little lean body mass as well. Even this small amount will help increase your metabolism so that your body will burn more fat even at rest.

You can learn the basics of weight lifting easily from a good book or an exercise video. If you want personal guidance, check with your local health club to see if it has trainers. Be sure to ask about academic qualifications, certification from organizations such as NSCA, and references from satisfied customers.

Change: You Got to Go with the Flow

If you were stranded alone on a desert island, which would your first priority be: (a) build a boat to escape in or (b) build a hut to live in?

If you chose (b), you're a survivor. Survivors don't struggle against bad situations. They adapt to them, even thrive in them.

That's the lesson Al Siebert, Ph.D., learned from interviewing people who went through terrible calamities and lived to tell their stories. They survived shipwrecks on high seas. Trapped on mountaintops, they endured days of withering cold. They wandered lost and alone through dark tropical rain forests. In every case, it was the same basic skill that kept them alive: adaptability.

"It wasn't this mythical individual against the sea, the mountain, or the elements. It was the individual *with* the sea, individual *with* the elements. They didn't fight their situations, they adapted to them and thrived," says Dr. Siebert, a semi-retired adjunct professor at Portland State University in Oregon and author of *The Survivor Personality* and *The Adult Student's Guide to Survival and Success.*

So what's the point? Few of us will ever have to harrow an arctic wilderness or find food in a desert. Most of the changes we encounter are far more ordinary: a shake-up at work, for example, or new neighbors or a divorce. But we can still learn from those people who experienced change in the extreme. That's important because, large or small, change is the one thing that none of us can avoid.

An Ever-Changing World

Not all change is sad or difficult. Often it can be happy and rewarding, such as when you have a baby or get promoted. But for some, especially as you get older, it may seem threatening.

"Perhaps people are afraid of change because they don't know where change is going to take them. They may be afraid that there is nothing to fall back on, and the unknown can be scary," says Peggy A. Stock, Ed.D., president of Westminster College in Salt Lake City and a lecturer on change. "Sometimes it just seems safer to stick with what we know."

Safe or not, the benefits of adapting far outweigh the risks. It helps you to cope with what

WOMEN ASK WHY

Why am I dumber than a 6-year-old when it comes to working with the Internet?

The answer is: You're not. Children aren't smarter when it comes to technology and the Internet; they just approach it differently from the way you do.

Children have two advantages over adults when it comes to using computers. First, they grew up with computers. A 6-year-old has never known a world without Web addresses and browsers and laptops. Navigating the Internet seems as natural to her as finding her way around a playground. Think back to something that you knew as a child but your parents didn't. You probably seemed like a whiz kid to them, too.

Second, kids aren't afraid of breaking things, including computers. You, on the other hand, probably view a computer as a complicated machine—and an investment of several thousand dollars. You tremble with the thought that pressing a wrong button could send that money up in a wisp of cybersmoke. Once you realize that it is practically impossible to actually break a computer by typing on your keyboard or clicking your mouse, you'll lose your fear and feel confident enough to play around on the 'net.

Expert consulted
Alan I. Marcus
Professor of history and a specialist in the history of technology
Iowa State University
Ames

is happening in the moment. The person who resists change will be out of sync with the rest of the world, Dr. Siebert says, and that's no fun. Being out of step with the people and the world around you may lead to a sense of isolation, helplessness, and a feeling that life has gone ahead without you.

Rather than focus on the risks of change, think about the opportunities it offers. An unexpected and even seemingly negative event can send your life in a positive direction, down a path you might otherwise have never traveled.

One man, whom Dr. Siebert interviewed, had been working for the same state agency for 20 years, when he was suddenly reassigned to another department, then another and another for the next 6 years. Instead of fighting or resenting the transfers, he accepted them as challenging opportunities and decided to learn his new jobs with enthusiasm.

He soon became integral to his new department, acquired valuable expertise about his agency, and jumped up three pay grades. "If you perceive change as a learning challenge, you'll take advantage of your situation and thrive. The people who remain resilient in life and increase their longevity are those who approach change with curiosity. They experiment and explore like playful children," Dr. Siebert says.

Easier said than done, of course. Even people who experience good change, such as buying their dream house or getting married, report increased stress and strain in their lives, Dr. Siebert says. So here are some guidelines to make navigating through a changing world just a little easier.

Revisit your successes. Think back to all the changes you have successfully handled in the past: getting married, having children, moving, starting a new job. Doing so will remind you how often you have triumphed over change. "You'll remember how well you coped and know that you'll handle this situation just as well," Dr. Siebert says.

Talk it over. In his work with women in their forties who have gone back to college, Dr. Siebert learned that they found it extremely reassuring and helpful to talk to other women in similar situations. Find other people who are going through or who have gone through a similar change, he recommends. They can give you advice or just give you peace of mind in knowing that you are not alone.

Stay ahead of the curve. If you see change on the horizon, don't react to it impulsively. Instead, be prepared for it. If it's at work, for example, learn new skills so that you can change careers, if you need to, or make yourself more valuable at your current job, says Dr. Siebert. "If you tell yourself, 'I have to learn all this to be competitive in today's world,' you won't resist the change. But if you're being told you have to do something in order to survive, you'll experience more distress," he says, "and react like a victim instead of a thriver."

Change for the fun of it. Get yourself used to change by making some enjoyable changes on your own accord, Dr. Stock suggests. Try a new sport such as inline skating or golf, read a new genre of books, find

KEEPING UP WITH THE TECHIES

If technology opens up a whole new world, it also opens up a whole new language. This new vocabulary leaves many people feeling lost and confused, says Larry Rosen, Ph.D., professor of psychology at California State University, Dominguez Hills, and coauthor of *TechnoStress: Coping with Technology @ Work @ Home @ Play.*

But just like any other language, you can learn a few key phrases or words to help you communicate with this technological society. Here's a quick primer on some of the most common computer terms and what they mean.

- The Internet: A global network of computers that lets people share information and resources.
- Cyber- (prefix): A person, place, or thing on the 'net. Examples: cyberspace, cyberpunk.
- E-mail: Electronic mail sent over the Internet or an online service.
- World Wide Web: A collection of multimedia documents that are connected. Web documents can include text, pictures, sounds, and video.
- Browser: Software used to navigate the World Wide Web.
- Search engine: A Web site that lets you search the Internet by typing in a keyword or phrase.
- Web address or URL (Uniform Resource Locator): Usually starts with "www." The location of a specific Web site.
- Surf the 'net: Randomly go from site to site on the Internet. Not looking for a specific page, just looking to see what is out there. Similar to channel surfing with your TV remote control.
- CD-ROM: An acronym that stands for "compact disc read-only memory," meaning the audiovisual information stored on a compact disc that you play in the CD-ROM drive (CD player) of a computer. The drive is very much like the CD player you use to play music on your stereo.
- Spam: Not the meat, but unwanted e-mail. Usually junk mail via the computer.

a new hobby. "Change can be fun and rewarding" she says. "It keeps life interesting."

Changing at the Speed of Light

Technology. It can be a scary word. Computers get faster, more powerful, and more intimidating every day. They intrude into everything we do, from reaching a customer service representative on the phone to starting your car. They are in your digital alarm clock, your VCR, your answering machine, the automatic teller machine. Just in one day, the amount of technology you interact with is staggering.

Short of moving into a jungle tree house, there is really no way to avoid it. Technological advancement is one kind of change we are all stuck with. And keeping up with it isn't particularly easy or intuitive. Although we can be extraordinarily adaptable, technology poses a special obstacle for us.

That's because it moves so fast, says Larry Rosen, Ph.D., professor of psychology at California State University, Dominguez Hills, and coauthor of *TechnoStress: Coping with Technology @ Work @ Home @ Play.*

According to Dr. Rosen, throughout most of recorded history, technological advances usually took years—sometimes even decades—to develop, and then took even longer to gain acceptance. All that time gave people the luxury of learning, adjusting, and deciding how this new technology would fit into their lives.

Almost at their leisure, people could grasp the significance of the wheel, the printing press, the automobile, and the television set. But today's technology evolves so quickly that it has eroded away that buffer. People don't have the time to learn, adjust, and adapt to one technological wonder before the next one makes its debut. The result is that we feel intimidated, stressed-out, and fearful, says Dr. Rosen.

The Benefits of Techno-Change

Technology may pose a more daunting façade than other types of change, but it also opens up a world of advantages to us. Here are just some of the many benefits of going with the flow of technology.

New perspectives. Keeping pace with technology prevents your thinking from becoming stagnant. And "by doing something that is so cutting-edge, you get a sense of feeling young at heart," says Alan I. Marcus, professor of history and a specialist in the history of technology at Iowa State University in Ames.

Control. Adapting to new technology gives you control over important aspects of your life: whose calls you receive, when and where you want to work, and how you get your news, travel, drive your car, and protect your home.

Greater access. From new recipes to up-to-the-minute medical knowledge, important information from around the globe is at your fingertips.

Fun. In addition to computer games, technology enables you to make videos of friends, listen to music in your office, and find new ideas for hobbies and creative outlets.

Close connection. Phones, cell phones, answering machines, pagers, and e-mail make contacting someone near or far a breeze. You can send pictures of children or grandchildren via videotape or e-mail pictures. You can use an Internet videophone to see and talk with each other on holidays. "I remember as a child hearing that someday we'll have picture telephones. Well, that someday is now," says Ann Wrixon, president and executive director of SeniorNet, an online community and Web site.

New friends. Whether it is meeting people online or joining a computer class, using technology introduces you to people of all backgrounds and ages. That interaction with a variety of people keeps you active and energized.

Better use of life experiences. The 20-year-old wunderkinds may be the ones inventing these technological marvels, but it is the people 40 and over who know what to do with them. "People with more life experience are the ones who use technology in the most innovative and exciting ways," Wrixon says.

Tackling Technology

It may be good to keep up, but with everything developing so quickly, how exactly can you do that? Where do you go for information? Here are some tips to get you up and running with technology now and to keep pace with it throughout your lifetime.

Read the popular press. Many newspapers now have weekly technology sections that address what's going on and what you can expect, says Dr. Marcus. Popular news magazines such as *Newsweek* and *Time* also have technology sections. The mainstream press keeps things simple and doesn't bog you down in a lot of techno-speak.

Take a class. Public libraries, community colleges, nonprofit organizations, and adult education centers often run classes for people who want to learn about new technology, especially computers. These are often fun, cheap, and designed for adults. Take a class to learn something new or master a program that you already use. Make sure that

THE SYMBOL OF A TECHNO-FEARFUL WORLD

Like many technologies, the VCR is an overly complex machine. "The people who have developed it tried to put everything in it, and because of that it is not easy to do the two things we want it to do—play tapes and record shows," says Larry Rosen, Ph.D., professor of psychology at California State University, Dominguez Hills, and coauthor of *Techno-Stress: Coping with Technology @ Work @ Home @ Play.*

But why has the VCR been ordained the ultimate symbol of the older person's inability to use technology? Mainly, because the VCR is everywhere. Even major technophobes own a VCR. Also, the VCR is in your face. Unlike other technologies that are tucked away in an office, it inhabits the most frequented room in your house, your living or family room.

And that flashing 12:00 is a constant reminder of your failure to master this bundle of bolts.

Because each VCR is different from the next, there are no universal rules about how to operate one. But Dr. Rosen has a few suggestions that will start you on your way to conquering just about any of those little mechanical monsters.

Read only parts of the manual. Some manuals are so poorly written that they don't help much, Dr. Rosen concedes. To make it simpler, read only about what you intend to use. Don't bog yourself down with unnecessary information.

Tape pages to the machine. Photocopy or rip out the pages of the manual that you use most and tape them to the VCR. That way you have them handy when you want to do something, like fix the clock after the electricity goes out.

Practice, practice, practice. Most people wait until they are running out the door or they need to tape something important before they start thinking about how to operate the machine. In their haste, they do it wrong and become even more flustered than usual with their own bumbling fingers. Pretend your VCR is a musical instrument. By practicing regularly when success isn't critical, you will be ready to perform under pressure when you really need to.

the instructor speaks in terms you can understand, Wrixon says.

Practice makes perfect. Just like anything else, using technology takes practice. "You'll get it over time. You don't have to learn it all now," Dr. Rosen says. Whether it be your VCR or your automatic car keys, spend time tinkering with them until you get the hang of it.

Tackle one task at a time. Don't set out to understand the intricate coding of a computer program. You don't need to. Instead, handle one function at a time. "Break it down into small components. You don't need to know everything, just the specifics of what you want to do," Wrixon says. Learn how to send an e-mail, record a show, or access a phone mail message. Once you have mastered one task, move on to another, she says.

Set a goal. Establish a reason you want to learn a certain technology. Do you want to learn how to use the Internet to study your family history or learn how to use a camcorder to videotape your children? This makes learning more fun and gives you a sense of purpose. If you just set out to learn something because you have to, you won't be as motivated, says Wrixon.

Lease or borrow technology. If you are not sure you want or need a new gizmo, you don't have to buy it, no matter what everyone else seems to be doing, Dr. Rosen says. Many stores now offer leasing for computers and technological equipment. Or ask a friend if you can use her devices for a while. That way, "you can decide whether you really like it, and you don't feel the pressure to buy it until you know if you want it," he says.

Advancing in the School of Life

It's been said that the definition of middle age is when you're sitting at home on Saturday night and the telephone rings, and you hope it isn't for you.

By the time we've reached our midthirties, many of us have settled into lives we're comfortable with, which usually includes an aversion to shaking things up.

"People are afraid that if they don't follow the patterns they've established over the years, they'll become strangers in their own lives," says Maryann Troiani, Psy.D., a clinical psychologist with the Mercer Group in Barrington, Illinois, and coauthor of *Spontaneous Optimism*. But expanding beyond our cozy little worlds is just the ticket to staying young, she says. "The more open people are to new experiences, the more they learn, the more passion and energy they have, and the better their quality of life."

So why not take advantage of the many new experiences the world has to offer you? It's been said that it's never too late to be what you might have been, so give it some creative thought. You could take up a sport, travel, volunteer, paint, sculpt, meditate, enroll in classes, get involved in local politics, join a hiking group, become an activist, study astronomy, learn photography, forge new friendships, become a computer whiz, become a better cook, become a better version of yourself. The possibilities are endless.

"The secret to staying young is reinventing yourself with each new decade of your life," says Laura Barbanel, Ed.D., professor and head of the graduate program in school psychology at Brooklyn College of the City University of New York.

Seek and Ye Shall Find

So how do you find the passions that suit you today, knowing that at age 50, 60, and beyond you'll be able to put your energy into whatever matters most to you as time goes by?

If you're not sure where to start, follow these simple steps.

Tap your friends and family. Talking to your family and friends—especially your oldest ones—can help remind you of things that thrilled you when you were younger, says Dr.

WOMAN TO WOMAN
The Power of Puppy Love

Elizabeth Goldstein, 39, was a photographer in New York City a few years ago when she began to sense an internal void that her career couldn't fill. Experiencing recurring bouts of depression, Elizabeth sometimes felt as if her life lacked purpose. But when she began volunteering at a local animal shelter, she discovered the healing—and youth-promoting—power of love.

I have loved animals for as long as I can remember, although I was never allowed to have pets while I was growing up. My father insisted that it was too much responsibility, and my mother wanted to keep her house free of fur balls and muddy paw prints.

As I got older, I found myself grappling with a sense that my life lacked purpose. The years were passing, and in the end, I would be old and stuck with the realization that I hadn't made any difference in the world. I decided not to let that happen. It was time to make some changes.

I started by making one positive change in a small world—that of a homeless animal. I visited a local animal shelter and, at age 31, adopted my first pet: a shy, scrawny black cat. I loved her from the moment I saw her, but I couldn't stop thinking about all the other cats and dogs still caged at the shelter, waiting for someone to come and save their lives.

I began walking shelter dogs, grooming cats, and socializing the animals that had been traumatized by their experiences with unkind people. Soon I joined the shelter's foster program, in which volunteers take very young or sick animals into their homes, give them the care they need, then return them when they are ready to be adopted.

Eight years later, I'm still hooked, still volunteering. And it's given me a payoff that I never expected: I feel younger and more alive now than when I started. There's nothing quite as healing—and renewing—as giving and receiving love. Making a difference in these animals' lives has made all the difference in mine.

Barbanel. Early hobbies, interests, and innate abilities that got stuffed once you started raising kids or pursuing a career can be fertile ground for inspiration now that you have wisdom and maturity on your side.

Take a test. If you think aptitude tests are only for high school students in search of a college major, you're only half right. One research firm based in New York City, Johnson O'Conner Research Foundation, has been helping people find their underlying talents and interests for more than 75 years and has had hundreds of thousands of clients.

A typical test measures musical aptitudes, structural visualization, inductive reasoning, memory, the ability to produce a flow of ideas, and many other forms of manifested brilliance you may be harboring. Other aptitude tests simply help you match your skills with your interests so that you can begin to pursue those things that you're great at and love.

Since some tests can cost $120 or more an hour, you'll want to check around for the best deal. Your phone book or local community college's continuing education office is a good place to start.

Do it yourself. If you'd rather identify your passions on your own and a little writing doesn't scare you, take this three-pronged approach, says Dr. Troiani. First, jot down your best traits, maybe friendliness, honesty, and loyalty—the ones many of us take for granted. Then make a second list of activities that you enjoy, which may include baking, building, learning, and singing. Third and most important, reflect on what you'd like to be remembered for when you're gone and write that down, too. Now, look for common themes and patterns in these three items, such as creativity or a desire to help people. The result is a small but personalized list of avenues you'll want to pursue, she says.

Make it happen. Now that you have a vision of what you'd like to do, how can you make it a reality? Look around you to find out what resources are available. Investigate your public library and local bookstores to learn more about subjects that are new to you. Contact hospitals, children's shelters, animal shelters, and religious organizations about volunteer work. Call local colleges and universities for information about continuing education courses. Check out Web sites to find leads and to make connec-

tions with others who share your talents and interest.

And then, get moving, says Dr. Barbanel. There's no time to waste in our bid to turn back the clock.

LIFE EXTENDER
Get Some Culture

Here's one of the best excuses you'll ever have to go to the theater or opera: It could help you live longer.

That's the word from Sweden, where a large study found that people who frequently attended cultural events such as theater, museums, sports—even sermons—actually lived longer than those who didn't.

It's no surprise that great concerts, plays, and movies can be inspiring. But how could *Les Miserables* help turn back your clock? Swedish researchers suggest that the "vicarious emotional arousal" caused by these events might enhance your immune system and, as a result, help your body fight disease. Just don't watch too many violent films: The study's researchers noted that it might have the opposite effect.

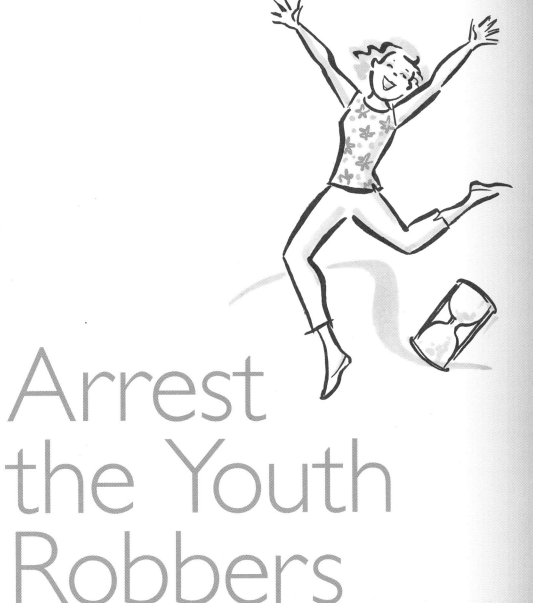

PART FOUR

Arrest the Youth Robbers

Defying Disease

Heart disease runs in my family. I'm either going to get it or I'm not. There's nothing I can really do about it."

Sound familiar?

Maybe heart disease isn't your worry. Maybe it's some other disease of "aging," like diabetes, cancer, or osteoporosis. Whatever the illness, it's easy to imagine it waiting like an unavoidable chasm in the road ahead. Genetics, as we know, are the blueprints of our lives. We believe they hold our fate, in the same way the ancients believed that fate was written in the stars.

Well, here's a news flash: Your fate isn't in the stars, and it isn't in your genes. You hold it in your very own hands.

"Certainly some diseases might have a genetic component, but the evidence clearly shows that other environmental issues—like lifestyle—play a key role," says Julie Buring, Sc.D., professor of ambulatory care and prevention at Harvard Medical School and Brigham and Women's Hospital in Boston. "Whether we develop a condition like cancer or heart disease, for example, is not something that's totally out of our control. There are many things we can do to reduce our risk."

What's more, it's never too late to make positive changes in your lifestyle—even if you're a fifty-something smoker who's overweight. "You may think that you should have made healthier choices when you were a teenager—and it's true that the earlier you do it the better—but we've found that even when elderly people quit smoking or start exercising it greatly benefits their overall health," Dr. Buring says.

The average 40-year-old woman still has another 40 years of life to look forward to. So start making healthy changes now, and you'll feel as good—or even better—throughout the second half of your life as you felt through the first.

Disease-Proof Your Lifestyle

Thanks to the men and women in white lab coats who've done countless hours of research, we now know that there are specific preventive measures we can take to lower our risk for many diseases as we age. Here are 10 key things you can start doing right away to help keep you healthy and feeling young.

Toss the smokes. Lung cancer, heart disease, stroke, high blood pressure, osteoporosis. The list of age-related diseases that smokers are at higher risk for goes on and on. Not to mention the wrinkles and stained teeth that make you look far older than your years. If you don't smoke, raise your right hand and swear you never will. Then give yourself a pat on the back. If you do smoke—stop. "Without a doubt, it's one of the best things you can do for your health," says Elizabeth Ross, M.D., a cardiologist at Washington Hospital Center in Washington, D.C.; spokesperson for the American Heart Association; and author of *Healing the Female Heart*. Within minutes of puffing your final cigarette, your blood pressure and pulse rate drop to normal. And after just 24 hours, your risk of having a heart attack decreases.

Add activity. Close to five million American adults say they don't do anything physically active in their leisure time. Now that's a lot of couch potatoes. And it turns out that more women are inactive than men. Everyone knows exercise is good for you—so why are so many women still stuck on the sofa? Perhaps you haven't found a fun activity that keeps you coming back for more. Or maybe you think you don't have the time. But it takes a lot less time than you probably realize.

"You don't have to go to a gym every day or become a marathon runner to get the benefits of exercise," Dr. Buring says. "The current recommendation for physical activity is something that virtually all of us can do." That's 30 minutes of accumulated moderate physical activity most days of the week. Walking the dog, gardening, housework—they all count.

Need another reason to trade in your recliner for a treadmill? How about 250,000 reasons? That's how many deaths per year in this country can be attributed to a lack of regular physical activity. In fact, regular exercise helps prevent everything from heart disease and diabetes to breast cancer and osteoporosis.

Control your weight. It's no secret that we tend to put on pounds as we grow older. A growing middle may seem like a harmless, natural part of aging, but it's not. "In this country, we gain an average of 7 pounds a decade," Dr. Buring says.

That adds up fast. If you weighed 125 at age 20, that means you'll tip the scale at 160 by the time you're 70. That rate of weight gain puts you at risk for a number of diseases including diabetes, heart disease, arthritis, and even gallstones.

Losing weight isn't easy. So your best bet is not to gain it in the first place. "Focus on maintaining your weight rather than trying to lose the extra pounds after you've already gained them," Dr. Buring says.

If you've already put on some pounds, try losing just 10. Even small reductions can go a long way in helping improve your condition if you have a problem like arthritis or high blood pressure, Dr. Buring says.

Pile your plate with fruits and veggies. That's right. One key to living a long, disease-free life can be found in the produce section of any grocery store. In fact, a study of 52 Italians aged 70 and older found that the healthy one-hundred-and-somethings ate more than twice as many vegetables as the younger folks.

That's not surprising since eating five servings of fruits and vegetables a day is associated with lower risks of several diseases, including cancer and stroke. And researchers have identified all sorts of healthy components in our produce. Not only are fruits and vegetables a natural source of antioxidants, vitamins, minerals, and fiber—they also contain phytonutrients like quercetin, lycopene, flavonoids, and ellagic acid, which are potential heart protectors and cancer fighters.

Eat a low-fat diet. Too much fat does a lot of nasty things to our bodies. First, it can clog up the arteries in our hearts and block blood vessels in our brains, putting us at risk for heart disease and stroke. Excess fat can also overstimulate our gallbladders and create the right conditions for painful gallstones. And of course, too much fat can make us, well, fat, which increases our risk for other diseases like cancer and diabetes.

Most experts agree that a low-fat diet should get no more than 25 percent (and preferably less) of its calories from fat. But not all fats are bad. The main one to limit in your diet is saturated fat, found in foods like meat, butter, and dairy products. Researchers say that the best way to cut down on saturated fat is to limit meat servings to 3 or 4 ounces a day, use little or no butter, switch to low-fat dairy foods, and cook with corn, canola, or olive oil.

Other fats to be wary of include the trans fatty acids found mostly in margarine and prepackaged snacks. They may be just as unhealthy for our hearts as saturated fat. You can cut your trans fatty acids by using trans-free margarine (partially hydrogenated oils are not listed as an ingredient) instead of regular margarine and by limiting the amount of snack foods you eat that contain partially hydrogenated oil.

Fill up on fiber. Eating a high-fiber diet may lower your risk for several diseases, including heart disease, diabetes, high blood pressure, obesity, and diverticulosis. And several small studies suggest that filling up on fiber can lower your risk of colon cancer. How does fiber protect against such a variety of diseases? For one thing,

WOMAN TO WOMAN

She Turned Her Health Around with a Simple Strategy

Sky-high blood pressure, the aches of arthritis, and 15 extra pounds gave 71-year-old Jennie Cargill of Cleveland Heights, Ohio, a powerful incentive to change her diet and beef up her exercise program. But as she peeled off the pounds, she got a bonus—it's as if she turned back the clock. Here's her story.

I was about 15 pounds overweight when I went in for my stress test. I had been dealing with a lot of family problems, and my blood pressure was already high. But I was about to find out just how high. The doctors put all these wires on me before I got on the treadmill.

"Well, let's get her reading," the technician said.

"It's 220 over 110," the nurse told him.

The technician hesitated. He said, "Excuse me, is that a blood pressure reading you're giving me?"

"Yes it is."

Well, after that, they wouldn't even let me take the stress test; my blood pressure was way too high. A little later, my doctor took me aside and said, "You know, we really have to do something about this." He knows that when he gets serious or acts concerned, I'll respond.

He immediately put me on a medication that would reduce my high blood pressure, and I was already taking a diuretic and another drug for heart problems. But I didn't want to rely on drugs.

Now, I've always exercised—we have lots of parks here—and I would try to walk at least 2 to 3 miles a day. But I de-

it acts like a sponge as it passes through our bodies, soaking up potentially harmful substances like cholesterol and binding to extra estrogen in the digestive tract, then removing them in our stool. Fiber also fills us up so we eat less.

The problem is that most people only get 11 to 13 grams of fiber a day—that's about half of the 25 to 35 grams experts recommend. To give cided I wanted to do more. So I started walking even faster. Before long, I could do a mile in 15 minutes. In addition, I signed up for a seniors' exercise class and toned and stretched my muscles for 1½ hours 4 days a week.

I also read somewhere that fiber helps fill you up. So I started eating a cereal called Fiber One and later switched to Post Shredded Wheat, which has less sodium. When I wanted to snack, instead of grabbing potato chips or something, I'd eat a handful of cereal and drink a cup of tea. Or I'd have cottage cheese and fruit, which I knew were low in fat and calories. And then for dinner, I would eat beans or something that would be filling along with chicken or fish.

To me, it's easier to eat this way. People would say, "Well, you should just go on a diet . . ." But I didn't want to go on a diet. I wanted a new way of eating. If you decide that you're not going to eat any pie or cake, then you just say, "I won't eat any cake at all." It's easier than saying, "Well, I won't eat chocolate cake, or I won't eat vanilla cake." Very simple.

In 4 to 6 weeks, I started feeling better. My clothes fit more loosely, and it seemed to help my arthritis. Suddenly, I could fly up and down the stairs. I'm not sure what helped me the most, but it was probably a combination of things. Losing the weight, the fish in my diet—these may help keep me limber.

My blood pressure came way down, too. The last time I was in my doctor's office, it was 134 over 82. And he was really pleased. He said to keep up the good work.

I told my daughter I'm going to live to be 100. I'm even reading a book now on how to do it. But that's not my only goal—I want to feel as great as I do now for the next 29 years.

your plate a fiber face-lift, add more foods like fruits, vegetables, beans, and whole-grain breads, cereals, rice, and pasta.

Supplement your diet. Our bodies need vitamins, minerals, and other important nutrients to function at their best. And if we all ate a low-fat diet high in fruits and vegetables every day, we'd probably get enough of these vital nutrients,

Dr. Buring says. But many of us don't. That's why it's important to take a multivitamin/mineral that provides the Daily Value for most nutrients. Think of it as an insurance policy for those days when our diet isn't up to snuff. But don't think because you're taking a vitamin that you don't have to eat a healthy diet, exercise, or quit smoking, Dr. Buring adds.

Another good reason to take a multi is the mounting evidence that supplementing your diet in this way may help you ward off disease. "People who take a multivitamin a day are less likely to have heart attacks," says Kathryn Rexrode, M.D., instructor at Harvard Medical School and associate physician in the division of preventive medicine at Brigham and Women's Hospital in Boston.

That may be because nutrients like folate, vitamin B_6, vitamin E, and beta-carotene have all been found to promote heart health. Folate may also help prevent colon cancer, cervical cancer, and strokes. Vitamin D lowers your risk for colon cancer and osteoporosis. Calcium may reduce rectal cancer risk along with preventing osteoporosis. Vitamin C and magnesium can help strengthen your bones and keep your blood pressure in check. The trace element selenium can protect a man's prostate from cancer. And beta-carotene has been shown to prevent cancer in lab animals.

With all that protection in a single pill, it's no wonder that one out of every two M.D.'s takes supplements or vitamins. "The benefits of taking a multivitamin are not absolutely proven," Dr. Rexrode says. "On the other hand, it's pretty cheap and safe."

Limit yourself to one drink.
While having one alcoholic drink a day may lower your risk of death, especially from heart disease, more than one may put you at risk for a whole host of other diseases including breast cancer, stroke, and osteoporosis, explains Marianne J. Legato, M.D., professor of medicine at Columbia University College of Physicians and Surgeons and founder/director of the Partnership for Women's Health at Columbia, both in New York City, and coauthor of *The Female Heart.* What's more, many heart specialists don't even recommend a drink a day to their patients.

"If they don't drink or they drink infrequently, I don't advise them to start," Dr. Legato says. "If they do imbibe, I tell them to keep it to one drink a day." So if you enjoy a good bottle of Lambrusco on occasion, pour yourself just one glass and recork the rest for later.

Get screened. Most women get a Pap smear once a year as part of their annual gynecological exam. But that's not the only potentially lifesaving test a woman should regularly have done. After age 40, a mammogram (earlier if there's a family history of breast cancer) and skin-cancer screening, for example, should also be included in every woman's yearly checkup. Later in this chapter, we discuss other health screenings that women shouldn't skip.

Know your risk factors. Many diseases run in families. So it's wise to know what that means for you. If a parent or sibling has had a condition like colon or breast cancer, for example, you should get the recommended screenings even at a younger age, Dr. Buring says. The same goes for breast cancer or diabetes.

WOMEN ASK WHY

Why are men encouraged to take an aspirin a day to keep their heart healthy, but women aren't?

In fact, some women with heart disease could very well enjoy the mild, blood-thinning benefits taking an aspirin a day provides. The problem is, we don't know enough about heart problems in women to make that kind of recommendation—yet.

Why? For years, most medical experts assumed that heart disease was exclusively a male problem. In fact, surveys showed that one out of three doctors wasn't aware that heart disease was the leading cause of death in women. Two out of three believed that women had the same heart disease symptoms as men. And an even higher percentage believed that if women do get heart disease, they do "better" than men.

As a result, relatively few female heart disease studies were conducted. But more information is slowly emerging. For one thing, we now know that women develop heart disease a little bit later than men. While the vast majority of guys are affected between the ages of 45 and 55, research shows that most women don't develop heart disease until after 55—a phenomenon attributed in part to estrogen levels.

It seems that estrogen helps keep your good high-density

No matter what your family history, you should have your blood pressure and cholesterol checked regularly. For cholesterol, that means every 5 years if your levels are normal. "Normal" is defined as having a total cholesterol of 150 or lower, with a total/high-density lipoprotein (HDL) ratio of 4.0 or lower. That ratio, which tells you how much of your total cholesterol is HDL, or "good" cholesterol, is a better predictor of heart disease risk for women than total cholesterol, HDL, low-density lipoprotein (LDL), or triglycerides, say doctors. If your cholesterol lipoprotein (HDL) cholesterol high and bad low-density lipoprotein (LDL) cholesterol in check. As you go through menopause and lose estrogen, however, your total cholesterol can begin to look more like a man's, raising your risk for heart disease. So much so, in fact, that by the time you're 65, your cholesterol levels could actually exceed those of a man.

For these and other reasons, some experts do recommend that women at greater risk for heart disease, such as those who have had a relative die from a heart attack, consider taking an aspirin a day. But if that's you, don't rush to your medicine cabinet just yet. There's evidence it may raise your risk for stroke or boost your blood pressure—obviously a problem for someone already suffering from hypertension. And aspirin has been known to cause stomach upset—as well as provoke asthma and allergies.

The best advice until we know more: If you're at risk for heart disease, get 30 minutes of exercise a day, eat less fat, find a way to relieve stress, and talk to your doctor about whether aspirin is right for you.

Expert consulted
Elizabeth Ross, M.D.
Cardiologist and spokesperson for the American Heart Association
Washington Hospital Center
Washington, D.C.

numbers are high, you should have them taken again in 4 months.

When it comes to your blood pressure, the American Heart Association suggests that you have it checked at least once every 2 years. An optimal reading is less than 120 over 80, and normal is less than 130 over 85. If you've had a higher reading, decide with your doctor how often you should have it checked.

"High blood pressure, which significantly raises your risk for stroke, is a silent disease. You could have it for years and not even know it," Dr. Buring says. "And you could be eating a healthy diet but still have high cholesterol, if it runs in your family. That's why you should have both your blood pressure and cholesterol checked regularly."

They are important to know because high levels are associated with increased risk of serious conditions such as heart disease and stroke, Dr. Buring says. If your levels are high, there are things you can do to lower them—like exercising and switching to a low-fat diet. In some cases, your doctor may want to put you on medication to help lower your levels.

Stop Disease before It Starts

As we grow older we start to feel, well, old. We may slow down a bit, and as a result, our bodies may slow down, too. Our joints ache a little more and our food is harder to digest. That's when disease prevention often becomes a priority in our lives, because we want to be as healthy and live as long as possible—aching joints and all. And it's true that the older we are, the higher our risk of developing certain diseases. But almost all of the life-shortening or slow-you-down diseases can be prevented. From dietary measures to early detection, here are the best prevention strategies for the most common diseases that affect women.

Arthritis

Arthritis. It's the nation's leading cause of disability among adults, and it's more likely to

BREATHE DEEPLY TO FIGHT DISEASE

Take a deep breath. Notice how your belly feels as if it's filling with air? Chances are you don't breathe that way most of the time, but instead take short shallow breaths that inflate your chest rather than your abdomen.

Some doctors believe shallow breathing so deprives our bodies of much-needed oxygen that it can lead to disease, so they teach their patients how to breathe properly. As silly as that may seem, they claim it significantly improves your health and may even help you live longer—much like aerobic exercise can. Here, three doctors explain the connection between breathing and health.

➤ "The human body is designed to discharge 70 percent of its toxins through breathing. Only a small percentage of toxins are discharged through sweat, defecation, and urination. If your breathing is not operating at peak efficiency, you are not ridding yourself of toxins properly. If less than 70 percent of your toxins are being released through breathing, other systems of your body, such as your kidneys, must work overtime. This overwork can set the stage for a number of illnesses," writes Gay Hendricks, Ph.D., a psychologist, in his book *Conscious Breathing*.

➤ "Breathing is unquestionably the single most important thing you do in your life. And breathing *right* is unquestionably the single most important thing you can do to *improve* your life. If you're interested in preventing illness, proper breathing may help you protect against angina, heart disease, respiratory infections, and fibromyalgia. It will also help you live a longer, more energetic, and stress-free life," writes Sheldon Saul Hendler, M.D., Ph.D., a doctor specializing in internal medicine, in his book *The Oxygen Breakthrough*.

➤ "Proper oxygen delivery to all parts of your body is crucial to health and well-being. . . . Breathing is the process by which oxygen enters the bloodstream, via the lungs. Thus, proper breathing, and correcting common breathing disorders, is the ultimate form of aerobics," writes Robert Fried, Ph.D., a psychology professor, in his book *The Breath Connection*.

So if you want to breathe easy about your health, try breathing deeply. It just might work.

strike women than men. At least 26 million women in the United States have some type of arthritis. The most common type—osteoarthritis—tends to occur more often in older people, usually striking between the ages of 45 and 65. That's because the cartilage around our joints can get worn down from years of wear and tear. Without cartilage to cushion them, bones rub together and cause pain, stiffness, and swelling. Several areas are particularly vulnerable, including the knees, hips, wrists, fingers, toes, neck, and lower back.

Many people may have osteoarthritis and not realize it because they have no symptoms, says Yvonne Sherrer, M.D., director of clinical research at the Center for Rheumatology, Immunology, and Arthritis in Fort Lauderdale, Florida. That's probably because certain lifestyle factors, which we describe below, can prevent symptoms from ever occurring. Here are the key actions experts recommend to keep osteoarthritis—or at least its symptoms—from bothering your bones.

Shed a few pounds. The more you weigh, the more stress certain joints have to bear. And the more stress you place on your joints, the more wear and tear that occurs. It just makes sense. "We know that if you keep your weight down to ideal body weight, then you're less likely to have problems with osteoarthritis of the knees," Dr. Sherrer says. If you are overweight, just losing 10 to 20 pounds can substantially reduce your risk of developing osteoarthritis symptoms, she says.

Get some exercise. Strong muscles equal healthier joints. That's because if your muscles are weak, they cannot effectively protect the joint they surround and may eventually cause it to slip out of alignment, explains Dr. Sherrer. As a result, certain areas of the joint may sustain a lot of pressure. But regular exercise increases your muscle strength, which helps adequately protect the joints and makes them more flexible. Activities that don't put a lot of stress on the joints, like walking and swimming, are best.

Don't overexercise. Serious athletes are more prone to osteoarthritis because they tend to overuse their joints. That speeds up the wear-and-tear process, Dr. Sherrer says. "If you abuse your joints, then you pay a price," she says. "And athletes are the most notorious group when it comes to overstressing the joints."

Cancer

Cancer is the second leading cause of death in this country. In 1999 alone it is estimated that 272,000 women will die from cancer. More than half of those deaths will be from lung, breast, and colorectal cancers.

Our risk for cancer increases as we grow older. Take colorectal cancer, for example. One in 150 women ages 40 to 59 developed this type of cancer from 1993 to 1995. Raise the age to 60 to 79 years, and the ratio jumps to 1 in 32.

"There's a very dramatic increase with age for most adult cancers," says Demetrius Albanes, M.D., senior investigator in the Cancer Prevention Studies Branch at the National Cancer Institute in Bethesda, Maryland. Scientists are not sure why cancer is largely an older person's disease, he says, but they theorize that it takes many

years of exposure to a variety of carcinogens to eventually cause the genetic damage that results in cancer. And they think that the weakening of our internal defenses as we grow older may also play a part in the disease.

There's at least one common type of cancer that is an exception to the aging rule and that's melanoma, a potentially deadly type of skin cancer. "Melanoma is actually a disease of young people," says Jessica Fewkes, M.D., assistant professor of dermatology at Harvard Medical School. "If you look at the largest group, the median age is around 40."

Whether you're 30, 40, or 60, you can take steps to lower your risk for any type of cancer. The most important thing you can do is obvious—don't smoke. Lighting up is to blame for up to 90 percent of all lung cancer cases—and lung cancer kills about 25,000 more women a year than breast cancer. If you do smoke, quitting now can dramatically lower your risk. Five years after kicking the habit, an ex-smoker's risk of dying from lung cancer decreases by about half. And after 10 smoke-free years, the risk is similar to that of a nonsmoker.

Keeping your weight within a healthy range and eating a diet that's low in dietary fat can also help lower your risk for lung, breast, and colon cancer, Dr. Albanes says. So can exercising regularly, he adds. In fact, a study of more than 1,800 women found that those who were moderately active had a 50 percent lower risk of breast cancer. Women who did more vigorous activity like swimming or running at least once a week were 80 percent less likely to develop breast cancer than inactive women.

Whether or not cancer runs in your family, you can further cut your cancer risk with these preventive measures.

Follow the five-a-day rule. When you sit down at your next meal, remember this catchy phrase: The food on your plate determines your fate. It may sound like a bit of a cliché, but research backs it up.

An analysis of more than 200 studies shows that a diet high in agricultural produce cuts your cancer risk in half. Consuming lots of fruits and vegetables can help prevent all three of the top cancer killers—lung, breast, and colon cancer, Dr. Albanes says. Researchers don't think there's just one component in produce that protects against cancer, but rather a bunch of components—such as the beta-carotene found in sweet potatoes and carrots, the vitamin C in green peppers and citrus fruit, and phytonutrients like the isothiocyanates found in broccoli. To improve your chances of staying cancer-free, aim for at least five fruits and vegetables a day.

Go for fiber. Perhaps you've heard that fiber may not be as beneficial in warding off colon cancer as was once thought. That's based on the findings from a study of nearly 89,000 nurses who got most of their fiber from fruits and vegetables but ate very little of the wheat bran fiber that many other studies have found prevents colon cancer. More research is being done to confirm the benefits of fiber, but until then, keep in mind that even the authors of the study involving the nurses say it's very important to stick with a high-fiber diet.

How might fiber help prevent colon cancer? By causing stool to move more quickly through the body. That's important because the less time harmful compounds in the stool stay in the colon, the less likely they are to do damage.

Eating a high-fiber diet may also help cut your risk for breast cancer. That's because fiber routinely binds to estrogen in the digestive tract and removes it from the body, Dr. Albanes explains. The less estrogen women are exposed to over their lifetimes, the lower their risk of breast cancer.

Pass up charred food. A survey of more than 900 women found that those who often ate well-cooked meat such as hamburger, beefsteak, and bacon were nearly five times more likely to develop breast cancer than women who preferred their meat rare to medium. Researchers say that may have been a result of exposure to cancer-causing compounds called heterocyclic amines, which form when meat and fish are cooked at high temperatures. You may be able to lower your risk of breast cancer by taking that steak off the grill before the black, crispy edges form.

Take a multi. There's some evidence that higher intakes of the trace mineral selenium and several vitamins such as A and E, along with some carotenoids, like beta-carotene may lower your risk for cancer, Dr. Albanes says. "We're also looking closely at dietary folate," he adds. And at least one study of 930 people suggests that taking extra calcium may help prevent colon cancer. While there isn't really strong evidence yet, it wouldn't hurt to take a multivitamin/mineral supplement every day.

Wear sunscreen. Unless you work on a submarine, you're bound to spend some time in the sun. The best thing that you can do to protect your skin from the sun's harmful rays is to wear sunscreen. "I recommend sunscreen with an SPF (sun protection factor) of at least 15 and full UVB/UVA protection," Dr. Fewkes says. And if you're going to be outside for a while, you should reapply the sunscreen every 2 to 3 hours, she adds.

Get tested. Cancer's a mysterious disease. You can do everything right from not smoking to eating a healthy diet and still find a lump that turns out to be malignant. Perhaps that's because the disease often has a genetic component—especially when it comes to melanoma, breast cancer, and colon cancer. Since you can't lower your cancer risk 100 percent, it's important to undergo screenings that can detect a tumor before you even have symptoms—when the cancer is most curable.

To help detect breast cancer in its earliest stages, women should have a yearly mammogram starting in their forties and should do self-exams every month, according to the National Cancer Institute. They should also have a clinical breast exam as part of their annual gynecological checkup. Some doctors suggest women begin getting yearly mammograms at age 50, but research shows that women under age 50 whose breast cancer was found through mammography had a 90 percent chance of survival. That's compared to the 77 percent survival rate of women whose cancer was found during a clinical breast exam.

To catch colorectal cancer—which is highly curable when found early—women over age 50 should have a fecal occult blood test at least every 2 years. An 18-year study by researchers at the University of Minnesota found that this simple test can lead to a 33 percent reduction in deaths when done every year. When the test was done every 2 years, the drop in deaths was 21 percent.

To head off skin cancer, you should see a dermatologist for a full-body screening every year if you're 41 or older and every 3 years if you're between the ages of 20 and 40. And you should also be on the lookout for any changes in your freckles and moles—it turns out that about half of all melanomas are found by the patient.

ALZHEIMER'S DISEASE: PIECING TOGETHER THE PUZZLE

Alzheimer's disease. Those two words strike fear in the hearts of many women. That's partly because until the 1980s we didn't know much about the disease. Now we do.

Many complex processes slowly occur in the brains of Alzheimer's patients. For starters, a protein fragment called beta amyloid builds up around nerve cells, forming dense deposits called plaques. Inside these nerve cells are twisted strands or tangles of fiber. In the regions attacked by Alzheimer's, some nerve cells die. Others lose their connections or *synapses* with nearby nerve cells. "Basically the brain is dying," says Claudia Kawas, M.D., associate professor of neurology and clinical director of Johns Hopkins Alzheimer's Disease Research Center in Baltimore.

More women than men develop Alzheimer's, most likely because women tend to live longer, Dr. Kawas says. The only known risk factors for the disease are age and genetics. "The risk of developing Alzheimer's doubles with every 5 years of life starting at age 65." And those with a family history of the disease have nearly double the risk.

There is currently no cure for Alzheimer's, but researchers are now focusing on three potential treatments.

The first is estrogen. A 14-year study of more than 8,000 women found that those on hormone-replacement therapy were 35 percent less likely to develop Alzheimer's.

The second uses nonsteroidal anti-inflammatory drugs like ibuprofen. In one study, people who took ibuprofen frequently had half the risk of developing Alzheimer's.

The third uses antioxidants such as vitamin E. In a study of 341 people with midstage Alzheimer's disease, those taking high doses of vitamin E were able to perform daily activities 25 percent longer. Supplementation of vitamin E also delayed entrance to nursing homes by an average of 7 months.

We probably haven't found a single cause or treatment yet because one may not exist, Dr. Kawas says. "Instead, what I think we're going to find is that Alzheimer's is like cancer in that there are several types of the same disease, each responding to different therapies."

Diabetes

Diabetes affects more than 15 million people in the United States—about 8 million of them women. And the majority of people with diabetes are age 65 and older. The disease becomes more common as we age for a couple of reasons. We tend to gain weight gradually over the years, and that puts us at greater risk for diabetes. And diabetes often goes undiagnosed for many years, making it appear that older people are more prone to the disease, but in reality, it's probably far more common among the middle-aged population than we realize, says Judith Gore Gearhart, M.D., associate professor of family medicine at the University of Mississippi Medical Center in Jackson.

People with Type II, or adult-onset, diabetes have elevated levels of the sugar glucose in their blood. This sugar buildup has two causes: either the body isn't producing enough insulin, which it uses to break down and utilize glucose, or the insulin is no longer doing its job properly. Oftentimes it's a combination of the two. Elevated glucose levels can lead to a whole host of complications, including blindness, kidney disease, and nervous system disease. People with diabetes also are two to four times more likely to have heart disease or a stroke than adults without diabetes.

There *are* key lifestyle factors that can significantly lower your risk for diabetes. The following suggestions from our experts can help you prevent the disease and the many complications that come with it.

Watch your weight. People who are overweight are much more likely to develop diabetes. "As a person gains more and more weight, they become insulin resistant," Dr. Gearhart says. That means the receptors in the cells that help insulin work are not sensitive to the insulin. The receptors are like a lock and insulin is the key—but when you're insulin resistant, the two don't fit. "Losing weight improves insulin sensitivity and helps tremendously with glucose control," she says. "In fact, many people are able to control their diabetes without medication when they lose enough weight."

Get moving. Regular exercise can also improve insulin sensitivity and can help you lose weight, Dr. Gearhart says. In fact, aerobic exercise almost immediately improves your blood sugar level and your insulin response—at least temporarily. And if you do it every day, it becomes a long-term effect, explains John Duncan, Ph.D., an exercise physiologist at Texas Woman's University Center for Research on Women's Health in Denton. That's why we recommend that people with diabetes exercise 5 days a week, he says.

Request the test. Diabetes tends to run in families. If you have a family history—or if you're overweight, have high blood pressure, high cholesterol, or any symptoms like intense thirst or frequent urination—ask your doctor about getting a fasting plasma glucose test, which measures the amount of glucose in your blood after an 8-hour fast. The earlier you catch diabetes, the earlier you can control it. "Many people have the disease for several years before being diagnosed," Dr. Gearhart says. "And as a result, they may already have organ damage."

Everyone age 45 or older should be tested, whether you have a family history or not. If the results of the test are normal, it should be repeated every third year after that.

Digestive Problems

A number of digestive problems tend to creep up as we age. One is diverticulosis, a condition especially common in people over 50, where the lining of the intestine bulges outward, forming tiny pouches called diverticula. These pouches are created by pressure that builds up from waste in the colon. The condition is usually painless, but if the pouches become infected, it can lead to a painful and more serious condition called diverticulitis.

Older people are also five times more likely to be constipated, and chronic constipation can lead to diverticulosis as well as hemorrhoids. And the over-60 crowd tends to have lower amounts of acid in their stomachs, which makes them more prone to gastritis (inflammation of the stomach lining).

Plus, painful gallstones affect about one in five people over age 65—most of them women—partly because the gallbladder may not contract as well when we're older, explains Melissa Palmer, M.D., a gastroenterologist and hepatologist in Plainview, New York. As a result, the stuff in the gallbladder that helps your body digest fat may form into hard stones, and they can clog up the ducts in the gallbladder or those that lead into the small intestine.

All of these digestive complaints can be treated, but there are steps you can take that may help prevent them as well. With these dietary and other preventive measures, you and your gut can be problem-free well into your seventies and beyond.

Get your fill of fiber. Eating a high-fiber diet can help prevent a number of digestive problems, including constipation, hemorrhoids, diverticulosis, and perhaps even gallstones. That's mainly because diets that are high in fiber lower the pressure generated in the bowel, says Susan Gordon, M.D., professor of medicine at MCP–Hahnemann University in Philadelphia. Experts recommend getting between 25 and 35

> ### LIFE EXTENDER
> #### *Slow Heart—Long Life*
>
> The express aisle. Fast food. Speed dial. In today's frantically paced world, quick often equals quality. But when it comes to longevity, it turns out slower is better. Research shows women who have slower hearts live longer.
>
> A study of more than 7,000 French women found that those with lower resting heart rates were less likely to die of almost any cause than those with higher heart rates. What's the best way to slow down a fast heart? With regular aerobic exercise, experts say. Just make sure to see a doctor before starting any exercise program.

grams of fiber a day. Try spreading out your fiber intake by eating foods like raisin bran, oatmeal, a sandwich on whole-wheat bread, broccoli, or an apple at every meal. Or you can take psyllium, which is a natural fiber supplement such as Metamucil, she says.

Flush out your pipes. Another way to lower pressure in the bowel is to drink enough fluids. "You need adequate fluids for proper bowel function in general," Dr. Gordon says. "And for fiber to work properly, you need adequate fluid in the bowel." A good rule of thumb is to drink at least eight 8-ounce glasses of fluids like water and juices every day. But beverages that contain caffeine or alcohol actually make you lose more fluids than you take in because of their diuretic effect. So don't count them toward your eight a day.

Lose weight slowly. Women who are overweight are more prone to getting gallstones, Dr. Gordon says. But losing weight too quickly can also put you at risk for developing the painful stones. So can yo-yo dieting, which is when you frequently lose weight and gain it back. That's one reason doctors recommend losing no more than 1 to 2 pounds a week.

Get off the couch. Physical activity can help keep you regular. Exercise gives your metabolism a boost, increases blood flow to the bowel, and helps the wastes move through your body faster, Dr. Gordon says.

Check your meds. If you frequently take aspirin or nonsteroidal anti-inflammatory drugs like Advil for arthritis or another condition, you may be putting yourself at risk for digestive problems. These drugs—when taken every day—can sometimes injure the stomach, which can lead to chronic conditions like gastritis and ulcers, Dr. Gordon says. If cutting back on the drugs isn't an option, taking enteric-coated pills can help, but it won't eliminate the risk, Dr. Palmer says.

Heart Disease and Stroke

Ask most people what the leading cause of death is for women, and they'll probably say breast cancer. Good guess, but it's wrong. Heart disease is the number one killer of both men *and* women in this country. In fact, a woman's risk of dying from a heart attack is five times greater than that of dying from breast cancer.

Most women are unaware of their heart disease risk because they think it's a man's disease—as did many doctors for a long time, Dr. Ross says. The focus has probably been on men because they tend to develop heart disease a decade earlier than women, she says. "We think that estrogen may be what protects women before they hit menopause," she adds.

Stroke—which is like a heart attack that occurs in the brain—is the third leading cause of death in this country. A stroke usually occurs when a blood vessel in the brain is blocked, either by a blood clot or by the same plaque buildup that can cause a heart attack. As a result, part of the brain is starved of blood and oxygen, and the cells in that area die.

Heart attacks and strokes both occur suddenly, but the conditions that cause them take years to develop. For starters, artery-clogging cholesterol builds up slowly over time. We tend to gain weight gradually as we grow older. And most people with diabetes—which is a major risk factor for heart disease and stroke—are age 65 or older. High blood pressure, another major risk factor for both diseases, is more common in women age 55 and older. "Heart disease and stroke have a lot of contributing risk factors," Dr. Ross says. "And many of those risk factors become more common as we age.

Since the two diseases have many similar causes and risk factors, most of the measures you can take to prevent one disease prevents the other as well. Take diet, for example. Eating low-fat, high-fiber fare prevents both heart disease and stroke by keeping your weight and blood pressure down and your arteries clear. Controlling your weight—especially the pounds that tend to stick to your middle—lowers your risk for both diseases. And so does reducing stress. When you're under stress, your body produces chemicals that over time can cause your arteries and blood vessels to stiffen—and that sets the stage for cholesterol buildup, Dr. Ross explains. So find ways to destress. Exercise, take a hot bath, read a romance novel—whatever works for you.

There are plenty of other ways to head off heart disease and stroke. Here are more strategies to help disease-proof both your heart and brain.

Kick the habit. The experts we talked to said the most important thing women can do to cut their risk for heart disease is to quit smoking—or better yet—never to start in the first place. "You quit smoking today, and your risk of heart disease goes down by tomorrow," Dr. Ross says. "Patients always say the damage has already been done, so it won't matter if they quit. It absolutely matters." Within 3 months of quitting, your circulation improves. After a year, your heart disease risk is half that of a smoker. And by 15 years, your risk is the same as that of a nonsmoker.

Smoking is a risk factor for stroke as well. In fact, it's probably the second highest risk factor after high blood pressure, Dr. Rexrode says. That's because smoking constricts blood vessels, speeds up the formation of plaque deposits, and makes it easier for blood clots to form. So putting out that cigarette for good will benefit both your heart *and* your head.

Find time to get physical. Regular exercise prevents heart disease and stroke in a number of ways. For starters, physical activity lowers blood pressure and stress levels and improves cholesterol by raising HDL levels. It also helps you to stay slim. Aerobic exercises, such as brisk walking, cycling, and swimming, help keep your cardiovascular system in great shape. "Exercise tackles all those things that put us at risk for heart disease and stroke," Dr. Ross says.

Mind your peas and cantaloupes. Fruits and vegetables contain all sorts of heart- and brain-friendly compounds from antioxidants to minerals like potassium, which helps by lowering blood pressure, Dr. Ross says. In fact, a study of more than 87,000 nurses found that women who ate the most fruits and vegetables were 40 percent less likely to have a stroke than those who ate the least. And experts say that munching on at least five servings of produce a day is good for your heart, too.

Call in a replacement. Women who have used hormone-replacement therapy have a 40 to 50 percent lower incidence of heart disease, Dr. Legato says. Estrogen's protective effect helps explain why the heart disease rate in women greatly increases after menopause. Estrogen protects the heart in several ways. First, the hormone has a positive effect on cholesterol. It

keeps the levels of HDL—that's the "good" cholesterol—up. It can also lower blood pressure by keeping blood vessels relaxed and wide open.

"I think every woman should consider hormone-replacement therapy," Dr. Ross says. "One of the newest estrogen therapies may actually be protective against breast cancer as well."

Hormone-replacement therapy may help prevent strokes, too. In one study that compared long-term users of postmenopausal estrogen to nonusers, the women who took estrogen had a 73 percent reduction in risk of death from vascular problems—including stroke. With all of estrogen's possible benefits, women really should talk to their doctors about whether hormone-replacement therapy is right for them, Dr. Ross says.

Take some extra E. Antioxidants such as vitamin E can help protect your heart from the ravages of free radicals—harmful oxygen molecules your body produces that damage tissues throughout the body. Inside your body, rogue free-radical molecules cause cholesterol to cling to artery walls and clog them up. Vitamin E can help prevent the cholesterol buildup by getting rid of free radicals before they do any damage.

The evidence is so convincing that some doctors even recommend vitamin E to their patients. "I recommend that my patients take supplemental vitamin E, because it can be hard to get enough of in a low-fat diet," says Dr. Ross, who suggests women take between 200 and 400 international units (IU) a day.

As for stroke, the research hasn't clearly shown that vitamin E can prevent stroke, Dr. Rexrode says. "There are much more convincing data for heart disease," she adds.

Go nuts. Research shows that nuts such as almonds, walnuts, and peanuts can be an important part of a heart-healthy diet. A 10-year study of more than 86,000 women by researchers at the Harvard School of Public Health found that

LIFE EXTENDER

Get the Benefits of Wine without Imbibing

We've all heard the news about booze: One glass of red wine a day can lower your risk of heart disease. But for those of us who don't make a habit of uncorking the Chianti, there are still ways to enjoy the health benefits of wine—such as guzzling a glass of grape juice.

The flavonoids found in both red wine and purple grape juice help prevent blood platelets from clumping, so they're less likely to form clots that can trigger a heart attack. One study by researchers at the University of Wisconsin found that folks who drank two 5-ounce glasses of purple grape juice a day for a week reduced the tendency for blood clots to form by 60 percent. Just make sure you choose purple grape juice made from Concord grapes. Red and white grape juices don't have the same effect.

women who ate more than 5 ounces of nuts a week were about a third less likely to develop heart disease than those eating less than an ounce a month. The unsaturated fats found in nuts help to lower cholesterol and may be what gives the nuts their protective effect, suggest researchers. Nuts are also high in other heart-healthy substances: vitamin E, potassium, magnesium, protein, and fiber. So if you're a frequent flier, don't pass on the cashews.

Take care of your teeth. What's the connection between your teeth, your heart, and your brain? It turns out that the bacteria that cause gum disease can travel through the bloodstream to your heart, where it can damage the heart walls or valves, explains Dr. Ross. The bacteria may also cause the release of clotting factors that can trigger a heart attack or stroke, she adds. Common signs of gum disease are red, swollen gums and bleeding after brushing. To keep your gums—and your heart and brain—healthy, brush your teeth at least twice a day, floss once a day, and see your dentist regularly, she suggests.

Osteoporosis

Ten million people in the United States have osteoporosis—and 80 percent of them are women. The problem is, you may not even know you have the disease until your bones become so weak that a bump or minor fall causes a fracture. In fact, one out of every two women will have an osteoporosis-related fracture in their lifetime, according to the National Osteoporosis Foundation. Women are more prone to developing osteoporosis because the steep drop in estrogen at menopause speeds up bone loss.

Even so, doctors are sending the message to women that this is not really an illness of aging. "It has been said that osteoporosis is not a geriatric disease, but a pediatric disease—and that's largely the truth," says Stanley Wallach, M.D., clinical professor of medicine at New York University School of Medicine, codirector of the Osteoporosis Center at the Hospital for Joint Diseases, and director of the American College of Nutrition, all in New York City. That's because behaviors that lead to osteoporosis—such as not getting enough calcium—often begin in childhood. Still, doctors agree it's never too late to bone up on bone. Just be aware that the older you are, the lower your baseline bone mass will be when you start.

Even if you're no teenager, experts say these five strategies can help strengthen your skeleton.

Nibble the right nutrients. Eating a calcium-rich diet from the time you're a little girl is the best way to build and maintain strong bones, says Dr. Sherrer, who is also author of *A Woman Doctor's Guide to Osteoporosis.* But for many teens and young women, milk, cheese, and other sources of calcium are off-limits. That's because these foods are typically high in fat, and girls in our culture are concerned about their weight at a very young age, Dr. Sherrer says. As a result, they're not building adequate bone during their peak developmental years and end up putting themselves at risk for osteoporosis later in life.

Even women way past their teen years can benefit from getting enough calcium. You may not be able to *add* bone, but you can maintain what you have, Dr. Wallach says. The bottom line is that premenopausal women need 1,000 milligrams of calcium a day through diet and supplements plus 400 IU of vitamin D, which helps your body absorb calcium. Postmenopausal women need even more: 1,500 milligrams of calcium and between 600 and 800 IU of vitamin D.

Get active. Physical activity is another key preventive measure that should be started at an early age and continued throughout life. Regular exercise—both aerobic, like fast walking, and lifting light weights—not only strengthens and maintains the bone you have but can also increase your bone mass. As you build and strengthen muscle—which is attached to your bones—you build bone as well, Dr. Sherrer explains. Try to work in at least 30 minutes of weight-bearing activity like brisk walking at least three times a week. Other weight-bearing activities, which simply means that they require you to bear your own body weight, include running, dancing, tennis, even bowling. Swimming and cycling, on the other hand, are not weight-bearing.

Measure your bone mass. Women should get a baseline bone-density test somewhere around the onset of menopause followed by a screening about one year after the start of menopause, says Dr. Wallach. Doctors can compare the numbers then to see if you've lost (or have failed to acquire enough) bone. If you have a family history of osteoporosis, you should be tested even earlier. The typical test is called the DEXA, which is a quick and painless x-ray that measures the density of the hip and spine.

Consider using hormone-replacement therapy. Giving women synthetic estrogen once their bodies have stopped producing their own can greatly reduce the risk of osteoporosis. That's because women who aren't taking estrogen can lose up to 20 percent of their bone mass in the 5 to 7 years following menopause, making them more susceptible to osteoporosis. Hormone-replacement therapy helps by preserving the bone you have, and in some cases it can add bone, Dr. Sherrer says. As with taking any prescription drug, hormone-replacement therapy is not without risks—certain kinds of estrogen, if taken inappropriately, may cause a small increase in your risk for breast cancer. So talk to your doctor about whether hormone-replacement therapy is right for you.

Avoid the big three. Another way to prevent further bone loss is to participate in the social graces as little as possible, Dr. Wallach says. "What I mean by that is smoking, alcohol use, and excessive caffeine use," he says. "All of these promote bone loss at any age."

How much is too much? Any amount of smoking is detrimental—not only to your bones but to your cardiovascular system as well, Dr. Wallach says. One alcoholic drink a day is okay, but drinking more than one a day may weaken your bones. And when it comes to caffeine, more than three cups of coffee a day or the equivalent in cola drinks can cause bone loss. So stick to decaf.

Keeping Your Senses Sharp

There are two fundamental facts that life teaches us as we age: The dosage information on cough syrup bottles is entirely too small to read, and teenagers mumble so much that you can never understand them.

Either that or our eyesight and hearing are starting to go.

Keen eyesight and precise hearing are important to us—our senses, after all, are our links to the world around us as we beautify our homes, clarify our career goals, pursue interests that we may not have had time for during our twenties, and watch our children grow toward adulthood.

So it makes good sense to keep our senses sharp and youthful.

Hear Ye, Hear Ye

How old were you when you went to your first amp-shaking, rip-roaring rock concert? How often have you been startled by a blast of volume when you slipped on your headphones at the start of your daily walk or jog? Can you count the times you've had to raise your voice to converse with a friend in city traffic?

As we go about our twenty-first-century lives, the tiny cells in our inner ears take a daily battering from amplified sound waves. Add the racket from snowblowers or lawn mowers on the weekends to the relentless engine revs and brake screeches of city streets, and the "Sounds of Silence" that Simon and Garfunkel once popularized seem like pure nostalgia.

But even before life got so loud, our ears didn't necessarily age gracefully. Age-related hearing loss is quite literally an age-old problem. It just happens to be one that we think won't ever happen to us.

Perhaps that's why women rarely come on their own volition to see John W. House, M.D., president of the renowned House Ear Institute in Los Angeles.

"Quite frankly, it's usually the husband or the partner who makes an issue of hearing loss. He'll have been saying, 'You know, I don't think your hearing is as good as it used to be,'" Dr. House says. She tags along reluctantly, hoping to prove him wrong.

It's very tempting to pretend it's not happening.

Can You Speak a Little Louder?

Even though age-related hearing loss generally begins in a person's fifties, it may happen sooner if hearing loss runs in your family or you've been exposed to excessively loud noises.

Still, if you're like most women, compensation and denial may prevent you from seeking help, says Dr. House. "They'll say people are mumbling or not speaking clearly, or they'll blame it on noisy restaurants."

As it turns out, noisy places are some of the most likely settings for age-related hearing loss to rear its unwelcome head. High-pitched conversation noise and rattling dishes will steal the words of your companions, and distractions may make it difficult for you to rely on a defense mechanism you may not even realize that you've been using: lipreading.

As women age, a change slowly takes place in a certain region of the inner ear, the cochlea, when hair cells that pick up high-pitched sounds begin to deteriorate.

You'll think that you can hear, but you don't always understand, and that's because you're actually hearing only part of a word spoken, says Dr. House.

Environmental noise only compounds the damage done by age alone. And while some lucky people—including Howard House, M.D., John's father and the founder of the House Ear Institute—hear perfectly into their nineties, by the age of 65, one in three women will suffer age-related hearing loss.

CAN YOU HEAR THIS?

The first sounds you lose to age are the high-pitched ones, so it's an early-warning sign when the people around you seem to be hearing things that you don't pick up.

Here are some you might be missing.

- Conversations of people talking with their backs turned to you. (In face-to-face communication, you may be lipreading without even realizing it.)
- The telephone ringing. (Has someone gotten the phone before you realized anyone was calling?)
- Tea kettles whistling. (Did you have to walk back into the kitchen to realize it's tea time?)
- The tick of a watch. (Is the second hand moving even though you don't hear it?)

The most classic sign of age-related hearing loss is not being able to fully understand the words of a conversation, even though you can hear the person talking, says John W. House, M.D., president of the renowned House Ear Institute in Los Angeles.

Preventing Hearing Loss

Whether you can still discern every word of every conversation or you've already noticed some loss of clarity, there is lots you can do to keep your hearing sharp and healthy.

Shhhhhh. The most important thing that you can do to preserve your hearing is to protect yourself from loud noises, says Dr. House. Wear ear protection if you're mowing the lawn, riding in a noisy motorboat, or going to a monster truck rally, he advises.

Buy the CD. Fun as it is to go and see your favorite stars on their nostalgia tours, be aware that the volume at concerts has gotten no less ear-splitting than what you remember. "We've seen people who suffered permanent hearing loss from one exposure at a concert or disco," says Dr. House.

Be smart on the job. Habitual exposure to noise is worse than the occasional blast of jet engine noise you hear as you climb the steps to your commuter flight. If you work in an area where people routinely have to raise their voices to be heard, you're at risk. Wear ear protection, and wear it consistently, says Dr. House.

Target Hearing Loss Early

If you have a hunch that you've begun to suffer mild hearing loss, get it checked out. It won't keep you younger to miss out on conversations at parties, lines in movies and plays, and directions at work.

What's more, hearing loss is not only a sign of age. "There are all kinds of causes of hearing loss, and sometimes they are treatable with surgery or medications," says Dr. House.

Otosclerosis, the hardening of bones within the ear, is a condition that is 90 percent curable with delicate surgery, for example. Other mimickers of age-related hearing loss include Ménière's disease, which is treated by medication or surgery, or even a benign tumor on a nerve that lies within the ear. Even though such tumors aren't malignant, they need to be detected early. Besides causing hearing loss, they can grow, causing pressure on the brain.

Begin at the beginning. The best specialist to see is an otolaryngologist, once known as an ear-nose-and-throat doctor, or an otologist, a medical doctor who specializes exclusively in diseases of the ear. Don't start at your local hearing-aid store, recommends Dr. House. "You can always go back and get a hearing aid if you need one, but first you need to rule out other problems."

Test it out. Once you've been checked for potential physiological problems of the ear or other hearing-related health problems, you'll probably be referred to an audiologist, a specialist in the testing of hearing. You may take a test in a soundproof booth with special headphones while you use a device to indicate when you hear sounds of various pitches with each ear.

Don't avoid your first aid. Hearing aids have become smaller, more inconspicuous, and vastly more sophisticated than they were even just a few years ago. Many are digital and capable of filtering out peripheral noise, so they selectively amplify the sounds you've been missing and most want to hear, like voices, says Dr. House.

"Often, I'll recommend a hearing aid, and someone will refuse," says Dr. House. "They tell me they're too young. But are they willing to go around saying, 'What? What? What?' and missing half of what goes on around them?" It's hardly a strategy designed to keep you young in body and in mind.

Early use of a hearing aid can help people adapt better to their hearing loss, Dr. House notes.

The Eyes Have It

It may happen gradually, as you slowly realize that it's getting tougher to see which eyebrows to pluck until you back away from the mirror. Or it may happen virtually overnight, as you suddenly become aware that you need to hold the newspaper at arm's length to read the classified ads.

Our ability to focus reaches its peak when we're around 12, then declines a little bit with every birthday thereafter. By the time we reach ages 35 to 45, many of us begin to notice we're holding reading matter so far away that our arms seem too short.

It's called presbyopia, the age-related vision change that occurs as your once-flexible lens becomes harder and less clear, says John B. Jeffers, M.D., an ophthalmologist at the Wills Eye Hospital in Philadelphia.

If you've already noticed your vision getting worse, all is not lost. Here's what to do.

Take a look—close-up. This is obvious, but it bears repeating. Schedule an eye examination to review the health of your eyes and the overall functioning of your visual system. This includes tests for how well your eyes focus on objects, both far and near, and how well they work together for depth perception, says Robert M. Greenburg, O.D., an optometrist and optometric consultant in Reston, Virginia.

Don't make excuses, like telling yourself you can see okay so long as the lighting is bright enough or you're feeling okay, advises Dr. Greenburg. It is true that your vision may be sharper in the bright light of a sunny day since the pupils constrict and increase your depth of focus. But you also deserve to see well indoors, in the soothing light of your den, or when you're walking the streets at twilight.

Squint no more. If you find yourself distorting your face to clear up blurry letters, you're doing yourself no youthful favors. Constant squinting deepens the lines around your eyes, making you look older. Squinting in bright sunlight is no better. Wear sunglasses to help to preserve the smooth appearance of your face around your eyes. Sunglasses will also help to prevent cataracts, which can be caused by sun damage, Dr. Greenburg says.

SHADES THAT WON'T FADE: YOUR GUIDE TO BUYING SUNGLASSES

Sure, sunglasses look great. What star would go out without them? But if you're serious about saving your sight, protection should be your number one priority when you go shopping for shades. Sunglasses will help to stave off crinkly little wrinkles around your eyes, but more important, they have been shown to reduce your chances of developing cataracts. They may even help to prevent age-related macular degeneration, a devastating condition in which elderly people lose their central sight, leaving them with only peripheral vision, explains Wayne Fung, M.D., an ophthalmologist at the California Pacific Medical Center in San Francisco.

Lenses should filter out at least 99 percent of the ultraviolet light and be made of impact-resistant material. Make sure that the lenses don't have sharp, unprotected edges that could cut your eye in a fall or sports-related injury, notes John B. Jeffers, M.D., an ophthalmologist with the Wills Eye Hospital in Philadelphia.

Ideally, they should be optically ground and tinted a neutral gray or green to block the most damaging wavelengths of ultraviolet A and B light, adds Robert M. Greenburg, O.D., an optometrist and optometric consultant in Reston, Virginia.

It's unlikely that you're going to find quality sunglasses meeting all these criteria on the bargain rack at your local drugstore, Dr. Greenburg explains. A good pair of sunglasses with the features recommended above will cost you about $50. Don't get taken in by the brand-name specialty sunglasses, however. Just because they are more expensive doesn't mean you are getting more or better protection.

Specs on specs. A new pair of glasses or a specially designed pair of contact lenses will restore your ability to see close-up again. Your own best option may be bifocals, bifocal contact lenses, or a pair of reading glasses. Check with your eye professional to see what she recommends.

Eyes Need Exercise

Although not all eye professionals agree, some advocate exercising the muscles in the eyes the same way you exercise the other muscles in your body. Dr. Greenburg suggests these tips for women who want to keep their visual system functioning well.

Keep track. As you go about your daily life, practice tracking moving objects and following things. Computer games help with this, but take frequent breaks.

Be shifty-eyed. Shift your gaze often. Fix your sights on something in one corner of the room, then the other in a rhythmic way.

Look here and there. Focus near, then focus far. When you're reading, look across the room every 2 minutes.

The Life of a Visionary

The very best thing that you can do to keep your eyes young and your vision sharp is to practice prevention. Investing a little attention in your eyesight now will go a long way toward keeping it healthy in the future. Here's what the experts recommend.

Look for yellow, orange, and green. Wayne Fung, M.D., an ophthalmologist at the

SECOND SIGHT

Steamy romance novels. Sunday drives. Watching your grandchildren grow. All of these pleasures can disappear into the darkness of age-related macular degeneration (ARMD), the leading cause of blindness in people over 65.

ARMD affects the macula, located in the center of the retina, the light-sensitive layer of tissue at the back of the eye. Slowly, the light-sensitive cells in the macula break down, causing loss of central vision and making it difficult to read, drive, or perform other everyday tasks. According to some studies, women may be at greater risk than men.

But there's new hope. Recent research conducted by Stuart Richer, O.D., Ph.D., chief of the optometry section at the DVA Medical Center in North Chicago, proposes a whole new way to prevent—and treat—ARMD. Here's the new sight-saving plan, based on his research.

Get tested. When taken together, four common vision tests can uncover the earliest signs of ARMD, says Dr. Richer. Ask your optometrist to administer the four tests in his study: the Amsler grid (which checks for distortions in central vision); contrast-sensitivity (which tests ability to distinguish between different-size objects); low-luminance, low-contrast (which measures ability to see in the dark); and glare-recovery (which tests ability to recover from glare).

Also, tell your optometrist if you are postmenopausal and not using estrogen replacement; have heart disease, high blood pressure, or high cholesterol; use photosensitizing drugs; or smoke. You are at higher risk for ARMD.

California Pacific Medical Center in San Francisco, recommends that women munch on fruits and vegetables rich in beta-carotene. The beta-carotene is important for good eye health, and eating fruits and vegetables adds fiber, which is important to your overall health. Good choices

Make like Popeye. It appears that ARMD can be delayed, or even reversed, with large doses of . . . spinach. In a preliminary study conducted by Dr. Richer, men with the common "dry" form of ARMD who consumed four to seven servings of spinach a week bettered their scores on the Amsler grid, contrast-sensitivity, and glare-recovery tests. Spinach contains lutein and zeaxanthin, antioxidants found in high amounts in the retina. It's thought that they protect the retina, either by absorbing eye-damaging blue light or by preventing free-radical damage.

Sauté spinach in a small amount of olive oil, or eat it with a meal that contains some fat. Fat helps the body absorb, store, and transport lutein, Dr. Richer explains. Also, if you are prone to kidney stones, eat kale instead of spinach. Kale contains lower levels of oxalic acid, which may contribute to the formation of kidney stones.

Take supplements. If you can't or won't eat your greens, take an antioxidant supplement that contains lutein, advises Dr. Richer. Studies suggest that 6 to 12 milligrams a day can benefit eyesight.

Mind your medication. If you're taking a blood-thinning medication, talk to your doctor before megadosing on spinach. The vitamin K it contains can interfere with anti-clotting drugs.

Shield those peepers. Purchase sunglasses that block out all ultraviolet A and B rays, including blue light, advises Dr. Richer. "Blue light is the short-wave, high-energy part of the visible ultraviolet spectrum, and it has been shown to damage the eyes."

Stub out those butts. Smoking constricts the delicate vessels that nourish the eyes, increasing the risk of ARMD.

annual eye examinations during your middle-aged years will diagnose cataracts early, before they begin to significantly interfere with your driving ability, sports and hobbies, and reading, Dr. Greenburg says.

Don't let blindness sneak up on you. Perhaps the most important reason for regular eye exams is glaucoma screening. When pressure builds behind the eye, damage can occur to the optic nerve, which can lead to blindness. Since there are no symptoms, an examination is your only path to early detection. If you have suffered a significant eye injury at any time during your life, or if you have blood relatives with glaucoma, you're at higher risk for glaucoma developing during middle age, says Dr. Jeffers.

Protect your peepers. As you lead your busy, active life, make sure that your eyes have the protection they need. Wear impact-resistant sunglasses or safety glasses that protect your eyes from injury as well as guard against ultraviolet rays. Wear a wide-brimmed hat while gardening, golfing, or watching sporting events in the sun. And if you're a weekend handywoman, be sure to wear eye protection while you're swinging that hammer.

Entwine with twine. Dr. Fung warns against a common travel-related eye injury from an unlikely source: bungee cords. It seems that women stretch the handy cords tightly around luggage or across skis on their roof racks. If one end snaps loose, it can fly very quickly into your eye, doing significant damage, he says.

include papaya, mango, kale, Swiss chard, pumpkin, broccoli, and spinach, he says.

Check your chance of cloudiness. As your eyes age, the protein material in your lens may begin to cloud—subtly at first, like adding drops of milk to a glass of water, one at a time. Getting

Memory like an Elephant

Who ran for vice president of the United States in 1984?

Don't remember? At the time, she was the subject of discussion over nearly every dinner table in America.

Bet you remember now—her face, if not her name.

Our brains are like that: More complex and marvelous than the most powerful computer, and yet we can find ourselves with a familiar piece of information stubbornly eluding us, right at the tip of our tongues.

When you first want that piece of information, you send your memory looking for it among the tons of intelligence stored away in your head. If everything goes right, you have the tidbit you are looking for a few milliseconds later.

Of course, not everything always goes right. And it goes wrong more often as you get older because your memory begins to slow down with age. Many of us have firsthand experience of that irritating little phenomenon. The question is: What can we do about it?

Oh, by the way . . . Geraldine Ferraro.

What's Going On in There?

First of all, relax. Stop worrying about Alzheimer's disease and early senility. Minor memory lapses are common, expected, and easily mended.

We usually begin to experience a gradual decline in memory at about age 30, but we are talking a *very* mild decline, says David Mitchell, Ph.D., associate professor of psychology and director of the Center for Aging Studies at Loyola University in Chicago. "Let's say you make a grocery list, and if you're like me, you forget to bring your list, but you go shopping anyway. When you get home, you're not surprised to find that you forgot to buy two or three items. As you get a bit older, you'll forget three or four," he says.

Aging isn't the only problem. You also have a lot more information to sort through now than when you were younger, and each day you add more data into your memory. With so much to remember, no wonder you forget. "The brain is a finite piece of tissue. Most people in memory research assume that as your system gets more and more information, it will take longer to search," Dr. Mitchell says.

As if a brain full of stuff wasn't enough, you probably also have a life full of distractions and responsibilities. Stretching yourself too thin can also lead to forgetting. "This is a time where women tend to be divided between their jobs, their families, and sometimes even their parents, as well as friends and their interests. Because of all this, there is a tendency to forget things," says Carolyn Adams-Price, Ph.D., associate professor of psychology and chairperson of the gerontology program at Mississippi State University in Starkville.

Keeping the Brain Up and Running

The brain, just like a muscle, needs to work out to stay fit. By challenging and pushing the brain to reach higher and do more, you make it stronger. Studies have shown that animals put into an enriched environment with many opportunities for exploratory activity actually undergo structural changes in the brain, improving their abilities both to learn and to remember, says Molly V. Wagster, Ph.D., program director of the neuropsychology of aging program at the National Institute on Aging in Bethesda, Maryland.

But what may be a challenge one day may be easy going the next. Although mastering any new mental task gets more difficult as you get older (no one knows why), once you have completely mastered a task, no matter how difficult, performing it no longer improves your brain. "We tend to reach plateaus in life. We work at something until we are good at it, then we continue to do it at the same level. But as you continue, the challenge disappears," says Arnold Scheibel, M.D., professor of neurobiology and psychology and former director of the Brain Research Institute at the University of California, Los Angeles.

In order to keep your brain and memory healthy as you get older, you must constantly seek out new challenges for them. Here are some recommended by Dr. Scheibel that will really give them a workout.

Take a language class. Learning a new language especially targets those areas of the brain that enhance memory. "It is a wonderful stimulus to memory function," Dr. Scheibel explains. If you don't have time to take a class, try learning from audiotapes. Use them as you drive to work each day. "Just work on it a half-hour a day. You can make a lot of progress in a couple weeks," he says.

Make beautiful music. The combination of visual, mental, and physical skills you use playing an instrument invigorates your brain, he says. Music, like many creative pursuits, improves your memory and provides a wonderful expressive outlet.

Seek out the opposite. Work on skills that are the exact opposite of what comes naturally to you. If you are artistic, dabble in the logical world of math or computers. If you are verbal, test out your ability to express yourself visually in painting or drawing.

Calculate in your head. Dr. Scheibel refuses to use calculators or computers to do basic math. Why? Because he found that relying on these timesaving devices soon eroded his ability to do math in his head. Math calculations challenge your brain and keep your memory in good shape.

Switch hands. For about 5 minutes a day, try being a lefty if you are a righty, or vice versa. Write, punch numbers into the telephone, or play tennis with your nondominant hand. This exercise develops the opposite side of your brain.

GREAT MIND GAMES

Challenging your mind doesn't necessarily mean taking a correspondence course in rocket science. You can have fun doing it. Playing games and solving puzzles, for example, can test your memory, strategic thinking, and other mental skills. Here are six games that can help improve your memory and your mind, according to Carolyn Adams-Price, Ph.D., associate professor of psychology and chairperson of the gerontology program at Mississippi State University in Starkville.

- Bridge. It's a game that involves both strategy and memory, providing a total mental workout.
- Chess. Although more strategy than memory, chess challenges your brain by forcing you to think several moves ahead.
- Cryptograms. Dr. Adams-Price considers cryptograms one of the best games to work your brain. The puzzle involves a lot of thinking and problem solving.
- Crossword puzzles. Solving them stretches your vocabulary and memory muscles. Enough said.
- Tetris. This video game requires fitting various shapes together at a rapid pace. The game requires spatial skills, which is the ability to visually place objects together. Spatial skills get better with practice, but you don't use these skills often in everyday life. Tetris offers a fun way to get them into shape.
- Minesweeper. This is another computer game. You click on grid squares to try to avoid hidden bombs. Play involves a lot of logical thinking.

Surround yourself with interesting people. Dr. Scheibel compares keeping company with intellectually stimulating people to playing tennis. "The very best thing you can do is play with someone better than you because you strive to be better. It is the same thing with people. When you feel, 'Gee, I am just a little bit out of my class here because everyone seems so much brighter,' that makes you extend, and I can't think of a better challenge," he says. Join book clubs, take classes, form discussion and writing groups, or just hang out with people who challenge you in conversation.

Improving Your Everyday Memory

It's the little things that drive you crazy: Where did I leave those papers? What is that guy's name? Did I forget the bread again? What is her phone number? "In the grand scheme of things, they are minor lapses of memory. They may become more frequent and aggravating as you get older, but they are not necessarily a cause for concern," Dr. Wagster says. "It may take you longer to remember a name than when you were 25, but you'll probably retrieve it—even if it takes a few hours."

To keep these petty memory problems from building up into major headaches, try some of the following memory techniques.

Pay attention. You often blame your memory when you can't remember, but many times, it is just as much the fault of your attention span. If you are not paying attention, you are not giving your memory a chance to absorb and store the information, Dr. Adams-Price says. When you are introduced to someone, stop, listen, think about the name, and even repeat it out loud. Do the same when you make an appointment.

Make the unconscious conscious. Make a mental note of all the little things you usually do without thinking, Dr. Scheibel says. For example, if you can never remember where you left your car keys, every time you put them somewhere, stop and make a point of saying to yourself: I put my car keys on the tabletop. "It's a new way of thinking, where you have to reiterate each action that you perform," he says.

Locate with 'loci.' Keep your tomatoes in the bathroom? Sounds crazy, but imagery like that is the basis of an ancient Greek memory system called the loci method. In the loci method, you picture whatever you want to remember as being in a certain place. For instance, say you want to make a mental grocery list. Dr. Adams-Price says to picture the milk on your couch, the bread on your CD player, the apples on the coffee table. Then as you need to remember the item, picture all the things in your living room. As you remember the place, like the couch, you will remember the milk.

Link words with images. Many people remember what they see better than what they hear. So think of what you need to remember as a visual image. For instance, you meet a man named Richard, says Sandra Monastero, a licensed psychologist at Friends Hospital in Philadelphia. In your mind, picture your new acquaintance as Richard the Lionhearted. You see him in your mind as a lion or dressed as a king. It sounds silly, but it works.

Sing your ABCs. If you can't remember someone's name, start reciting the alphabet in your head. "Oftentimes you can cue yourself to remember the name when you come upon the letter it starts with," Dr. Adams-Price says.

Divide and conquer numbers. Cell phones, pager numbers, e-mail addresses, security codes—it seems the numbers you need to remember are infinite. All of those digits easily get mixed up in your brain matter. To make it easier for you, break them down in chunks, Monastero says. Perhaps your automatic teller machine code is 7241. Remember it as "seventy-

two, forty-one" instead of "seven, two, four, one." Divide it into two numbers instead of four.

Get Organized

If you are the kind of person who files all your important papers under "S" for "Stuff," you may be one of those people who loses everything from her car keys to her track of time. "Disorganization is part of the problem. People who aren't well-organized are more likely to forget where they put things," Dr. Adams-Price says.

The antidote is the same one you would use to cure a sloppy room: Straighten the place up. You can start here.

Invest in an appointment book. An appointment book can be your central location for information, Monastero says. Use this appointment book for phone numbers, schedules, lists of things to do, appointments, and everything else you need to know. By doing so, you take a lot of stress off your memory. Be careful to divide your book into as few sections as possible. Too many can be overwhelming and defeat your purpose.

Find the best of times. A study at the University of Arizona tested a group of younger people and a group of older people at different times of the day. The researchers found that young people performed better in the evening, while the older group tested better in the morning. It may be that your own circadian rhythms affect how well your memory functions, Dr. Mitchell says. While the study found that the morning was better as people got older, Dr. Mitchell advises you to figure out your own optimal time. "If you have a choice, schedule important things you have to do at that time," he says.

Place things where you will see them. Out of sight, out of mind, right? That's usually the problem, especially in forgetting to take pills,

WOMEN ASK WHY

Why is it that I can remember the details of my senior prom, but I can't remember where I had dinner last Saturday night?

For the same reason that just about anyone old enough to remember can tell you exactly what they were doing on the day President John F. Kennedy was assassinated: You have a "flashbulb" memory.

You form a flashbulb memory when you experience an event so significant that you repeat it in your mind for years and years afterward, until you freeze that moment in time.

If you were like many teenage girls, the senior prom—for better or for worse—was a defining moment in your life. For weeks before the big night, you may have painstakingly gone over every detail: your dress, your shoes, your hair, your jewelry.

Afterward, because it was such a significant memory, you replayed it over and over in your mind, probably so often that you'll never forget it.

As for last Saturday's dinner, what was special about it? It probably wasn't much different from dinner the Saturday before, or the Saturday before that. So why on earth would you remember? After all, it wasn't exactly a prom.

Expert consulted
Carolyn Adams-Price, Ph.D.
Associate professor of psychology and chair-
*   person of the gerontology program*
Mississippi State University
Starkville

keep your car keys on the table by the door; always leave your reading glasses on your nightstand. Monastero also suggests appointing a special location for the next day's work materials. "Have everything for the next day gathered together and put in a central spot the night before. That way, when the morning comes, you don't have to think about where you put things or what you have to do that day," she says.

Color your world. Bright colors help you find objects you often lose. Put your keys on colorful, large key chains. Place a bright-colored string around your reading glasses. With bright colors screaming at you, you won't have to work as hard to find lost items, Monastero says.

Make little ones out of big ones. A big project or an outrageous amount of material to remember can overwhelm you. That sinking feeling leads you to procrastination, which means that you end up doing an awful lot of work at the last moment—and inevitably you forget something. Instead of getting lost in the big picture, break up a large project into smaller discrete tasks, Monastero says. Tackle each task one at a time and complete it. This makes a project more manageable and less overpowering.

Do it now. If behavior guru and Harvard educator B. F. Skinner heard it was going to rain, he got up right then and put the umbrella up against the door so that he couldn't miss it, says Dr. Mitchell. The best way to not forget something is to act upon it as soon as possible, he says.

papers, and all sorts of important things. So leave them where you have to see them, Monastero says. Some examples: Put your medications inside your coffee cup, leave documents on your alarm clock. "Make sure that you have to move it to get to something else," she suggests.

Designate special spots. Get into the habit of leaving objects in designated spots. Always

Make lists. Put information on paper. It takes a load off your mind when it comes to remembering. Lists also force you to organize your ideas. "Even if you forget the list, you took the time to compose your thoughts, which will help you in trying to retrieve the information," Dr. Wagster says.

Living a Memory-Enhancing Lifestyle

Lest we forget, the brain is a part of the body. And just like the rest of your body, it needs the basics: good nutrition and exercise. If you are lacking in these areas, your brain—no matter how well-prepared—will never work at its full capacity. So here are some tips designed to help with the care and feeding of your gray matter.

Get up and go. Regular exercise will help your memory. It's as simple as taking a 50-minute brisk walk three or four times a week, says Robert E. Dustman, Ph.D., research career scientist and director of neuropsychology research at the Veterans Affairs Medical Center in Salt Lake City. In a study of 45 men and women, ages 55 to 70, researchers found that people who started a walking program scored better on visual memory and mental flexibility tests.

"It makes sense that aerobic exercise should be good for the brain, because it's good for the cardiovascular system, and that system is the gateway to the brain," says Dr. Dustman, the study's author.

Toss in strawberries and spinach. Both may help fight the effects of aging on the brain. Recent research shows that giving an extract from either strawberries or spinach to rats helps retard age-related problems of the brain.

"These do have a positive effect on slowing age-related cognitive decline—at least in rats," Dr. Wagster says. Although the findings have yet to be confirmed in people, she suggests that individuals eat a balanced diet, which includes foods, such as strawberries and spinach, that are rich in antioxidants.

Supplement with C and E. Because vitamins C and E are antioxidants, they are thought to protect your brain from the normal ravages of aging. Although you should get most nutrients from a diet filled with fruits, vegetables, and whole grains, you may need to add more of these important antioxidants, Dr. Scheibel says, so take a supplement of 400 international units of vitamin E and 1,000 milligrams of C a day. "The data are more and more pushing in the direction that these two protect the brain," he says.

Get enough of the Bs. The B vitamins thiamin, vitamin B_6, and vitamin B_{12} all play a role in keeping the brain healthy, Dr. Scheibel says. If you are not getting enough of these three B vitamins from your diet, try a good B-complex vitamin supplement, he suggests.

Without enough thiamin, your brain can't use glucose as well. And if that happens, your brain can't perform up to speed. You need at least 1.5 milligrams a day. Good food sources include rice bran, pork, beef, fresh peas, beans, and wheat germ.

Meanwhile, vitamin B_6 helps make neurotransmitters, the chemicals that allow brain cells to communicate. Take at least 2 milligrams per day, from either a supplement or good food sources, such as bananas, avocados, chicken, beef, or eggs.

Last but not least, you need vitamin B_{12} to protect the production of myelin, a fatty covering that insulates nerve fibers. If you don't get enough B_{12}, you may experience memory loss and confusion. You need 6 micrograms a day, either from a supplement or from food sources such as clams, ham, lamb, cooked oysters, king crab, herring, salmon, or tuna.

Sex: The Best Is Yet to Come

Wish you were in your twenties again? The Sex in America study, which polled more than 3,000 people, found that women in their early twenties reported the least amount of orgasms during sex, while women in their forties and fifties reported the most.

That's right, sex gets better as women get older.

Not only that, but the better it gets, the more youthful we feel. "Women are saying to me that this is a really special time in their lives, that they feel really young. Sex is something that is going to continue in their lives," says Louise Merves-Okin, Ph.D., a clinical psychologist and marriage and family therapist in Jenkintown, Pennsylvania.

But how can that be? Isn't everything supposed to get *worse* as we get older, to break down and fall apart? Whatever is *supposed* to happen, here are three areas of our lives where things definitely improve.

Our bodies. Teenagers aren't the only ones with raging hormones. Many sex researchers believe that because of a hormonal surge, a woman hits her sexual peak in her thirties or later, says

Karen Donahey, Ph.D., director of the sex and marital therapy program at Northwestern University Medical Center in Chicago. By then women also feel more comfortable with their bodies. They know what they like and what they don't like.

And after menopause, the risk of pregnancy is gone. "Many women feel more sexual after menopause because they don't have to worry about birth control," says Alice Kahn Ladas, Ed.D., a licensed psychologist practicing in New York City and Santa Fe, New Mexico, and coauthor of *The G-Spot*.

Our feelings. Women past their midthirties tend to be in a secure relationship, advanced in their careers, happy with their children and home life, and generally more confident. When everything else is right in our lives, good sex often follows. "When we're happy with our lives, we're more fulfilled sexually," says Dr. Donahey.

Our circumstances. As we reach our forties and fifties, our family responsibilities fall off a bit. Children move out or are old enough to rely on us less. Now we can focus more of our emotional energy on our love lives. And for a lot of us, that's when the fun really begins.

Of course, not every obstacle to a good sex life moves out with the kids. Everyday life can have a way of getting between you and the bedroom if you let it. But with the right approach, you can keep the sparks flying for the rest of your life. Here's how.

Making Time to Make Love

After a day of errands, chores, cooking, cleaning, and working, sex may not even enter your mind, and if it does, you meet it with a groan. "I hear this more and more in my office. By the time people take a breather late at night, the last thing they want to do is have sex," says Adelaide Nardone, M.D., a gynecologist in Mount Kisco, New York.

As your workload and family responsibilities build up, something's got to give. Unfortunately, what often gives is sex. More times than not, nothing is wrong with your libido, but you run around so much that you're just plain tired, Dr. Nardone says.

So not to worry. Your sex life just needs nurturing. "You put time into things you enjoy. You try to be creative and make important things in your life special. Sexuality shouldn't be any different," Dr. Merves-Okin says.

Need a jump start? Here are some ideas for putting the passion back into your life.

THE BIOLOGICAL CLOCK: IS IT TICKING LONGER?

A woman gives birth to her first child at age 63. A California fertility clinic's *average* patient age is 48. Why are women waiting so long to get pregnant? Has something changed in the biological clock?

Actually, the clock hasn't changed at all. "It's still ticking on its own," says Faith Frieden, M.D., director of maternal-fetal medicine at Englewood Hospital and Medical Center in New Jersey. "But women and medical technology are pushing its limits."

A woman's body works the way it always has. Every month, during ovulation, she releases an egg that can be fertilized. This process continues until she goes through menopause, usually in her early fifties. As long as she ovulates, a woman has the potential to get pregnant.

The quality and quantity of available eggs, however, decline as she gets older, reducing her fertility. Only recently have fertility breakthroughs increased her chances of successfully bearing children later in life. "Women feel like they have more options, thanks to technology," Dr. Frieden says.

Also, women are healthier than their counterparts of years ago. They can expect to live much longer than their great-grandmothers did and remain much healthier through middle age, so many are waiting until their late thirties and forties to have children. In the meantime, many are pursuing careers, says Dr. Frieden.

Unfortunately, with later-in-life pregnancies, there are some risks. A study of 24,000 women at the University of California, Davis, found that first-time mothers over 40 were twice as likely to have a cesarean section and were much more likely to develop pregnancy-related diabetes and high blood pressure. "It is certainly possible, and it is most likely to have a good outcome, but these women should know what they are getting into," Dr. Frieden says. "Unfortunately, late-in-life pregnancies carry a higher risk of fetal abnormalities, such as Down's syndrome."

AGE ERASER

Sex: The Real Elixir of Youth?

Forget that trip to the skin-care aisle. According to investigators in Scotland, the secret to looking younger is right in your own bedroom.

Researchers at the Royal Edinburgh Hospital interviewed 3,500 people who looked and felt younger than they actually were. The survey found that these younger-looking people had sex at a "significantly higher" rate in both "quality and quantity" than the average person.

"Improving the quality of one's sex life can help a person to look between 4 and 7 years younger," says Dr. David Weeks of the Royal Edinburgh Hospital in Edinburgh, Scotland, in his book *Secrets of the Superyoung*. "This results from significant reductions in stress, greater contentment, and better sleep."

Pencil it in. In today's hectic world, nothing seems to get done until it's scheduled. The same goes for sex. "Make a conscious effort to set time aside. It may seem unnatural, but it works. I mean, a tennis game isn't going to suddenly appear. You have to make arrangements for it," says Wendy Fader, Ph.D., a licensed psychologist and certified sex therapist in Boca Raton, Florida. Write it into your schedule. Treat it as you would any other very important meeting, because it *is* just as important.

Set the mood. Light a few candles, grab a bottle of wine, put on a CD of romantic music, even dance with your partner in your bedroom. When you create a romantic mood, things often fall into place. Make sex a pleasurable way to end the day, instead of a chore, Dr. Merves-Okin says.

Wake up early. No matter what kind of day you've had, you're probably too exhausted by 11:00 P.M. to make love. Don't make sex a night-time-only activity, Dr. Nardone says. Get up a half-hour earlier and make love in the morning, or take a lunch break and rendezvous at home.

Attempt a 10-minute tryst. Take advantage of those few spare minutes you have here and there. "There are all kinds of possibilities for sexual interludes," Dr. Fader says. "A 10-minute quickie is just fine. They don't always have to be 2-hour marathon sessions."

Send the kids away. Call a babysitter or ask a relative to watch them while you enjoy a romantic weekend away or even just a relaxing, sensual dinner, Dr. Nardone suggests.

Think about it—all day. "When you wake up in the morning, think about sex. If you think about it all day, it is more likely to happen," Dr. Fader says. Build up a sense of anticipation, and you won't be able to wait until you get home.

Clue him in on your desires. Now that you're in the right mindset, your job is to get him on the same page. "Seduce your mate throughout the day," Dr. Fader says. Leave him love notes that suggest what he'll have waiting for him when he gets home. Or if you are really bold, try the art of seduction over the phone. "That will smooth the way to get the two of you together. It is very titillating," she says.

Tell him that you love him. Sex is the ultimate expression of your love for each other. Unfortunately, as your lives get busy, you sometimes forget to express that love. Without that overall feeling of caring and tenderness, sex often falls by the wayside. "The other person wants to know that you're interested in him and that you love him," Dr. Merves-Okin says. "Start in the morning by leaving him a note that says, 'I'm glad I married you.' Tell him, 'I love you,' every day and tell him the things you love about him."

Wear that little black dress. After a day in jeans and a sweatshirt, you won't feel very seductive. But put on a party dress or teddy, and you may find that looking sexy can make you feel sexy. "Even if it is just you and your husband, put on something nice. You'll feel like a woman," Dr. Nardone says.

Get in touch. Sex shouldn't be the only time you and your mate touch. Hold hands, hug, kiss, sleep in an embrace—every day, Dr. Merves-Okin says. Simple affection often evolves into a caring, wonderful sex life.

Take time *not* to have sex. Your kids aren't the only ones who need quality time with you. Take a walk or set aside 10 minutes a day where you ask each other how your day went. "Get a sense of togetherness," Dr. Nardone says. That sense of connectedness fosters a loving, caring atmosphere where sex can thrive.

Every Night Is a New Experience

A patient of Dr. Nardone, a forty-something single woman, came into the office one day, raving about a new love in her life, a forty-something man. She proceeded to gush that they were having sex twice a day—every day. Where did this middle-aged couple find their inspiration? In the very newness of their relationship. It had spark, romance, and spontaneity—the traits that lead to a great sex life.

What many people perceive as a lack of desire is, frankly, boredom. While spending years with the same partner generates an intimacy and closeness that can enhance sexual pleasure, it also creates a "been there, done that" attitude. "Anything that you do for 15 years is going to be

boring," Dr. Fader says. "Even people who say they have a decent sex life find that it is a pretty-mapped-out process. They do it the same way every time. It tends to be humdrum."

Don't worry, you don't have to throw out years of a good, established relationship for someone new to rekindle your sexual passion. In fact, combining your maturity and intimacy with newness and excitement will bring your love life to a whole new level. Making the commonplace new again will take a little creativity and time, but the results will be well worth the effort. Here's how to keep the bedroom sizzling.

Change the scenery. A candle here, music there, some flowers—all these small changes make it feel like a whole new experience. "I would begin with lighting a candle. Make it more inviting," Dr. Fader says.

Indulge in satin. Nothing says let's make love better than satin sheets. Luxurious, soft, and sexy, these silky sheets transform a plain old bedroom into an exotic locale, Dr. Fader says. Put them on when you want to give your partner a hint that tonight's the night.

Find a new location. Always have sex in the bedroom? Why not the kitchen, the dining room, the bathroom? Simply having sex in another room of the house can take it out of the realm of the ordinary, Dr. Ladas says. If you want to go beyond that, rent a hotel room or get away for the weekend and make love in an entirely new setting.

Please each other in new ways. For most couples, sex is goal oriented. Everything leads to one objective: orgasm through intercourse. That takes a lot of the fun out of it, says Beverly Whipple, R.N., Ph.D., professor of nursing at Rutgers College of Nursing in Newark, New Jersey, and president of the American Association of Sex Educators, Counselors, and Therapists. "I like to teach people to climb a 'staircase of pleasure.' Each step is pleasurable in itself and

WOMEN ASK WHY

Why are so many women attracted to older men?

Power is a strong aphrodisiac for many women, and older men often radiate power from the core. That doesn't mean power over the women who find them interesting, but the maturity and experience of many older men often give them control over many aspects of their own lives. Women who long for stability can find these traits irresistible.

Older men are more likely to have climbed the corporate ladder, so they are at a pinnacle in their careers. And unlike their younger counterparts, they're not questioning their life's purpose or career goals, or trying to decide if going to graduate school would be a good idea. Older gentlemen tend to be more confident and self-assured, and they have been around the block a few times, so they know what they want and how to get it. Their established, rock-solid, powerful nature is a definite turn-on to some women who yearn for stability.

In other cases, younger women and older men find themselves in the same stage of life. Say a woman in her late thirties wants to settle down, buy a house, and start a family. A man in that age bracket may not be ready to give up his career or his freedom yet, whereas a man in his forties who feels that he's accomplished what he set out to do in life may be looking for that very thing.

Expert consulted
Louise Merves-Okin, Ph.D.
Clinical psychologist and marriage and family therapist
Jenkintown, Pennsylvania

Learn what else your bodies like. Spend a day touching each other all over, from your toes to the top of your head. Try soft touches, harder massagelike touches. You may find that many other parts of the body—your ears, toes, and knees—can be sensual and erotic, Dr. Whipple says. These discoveries will generate plenty of new ideas for making love.

Reverse your roles. Are you always the seduced and he the seducer, or vice versa? Trade places. Playing the same role every time during lovemaking can become just as much of a rut as doing it in the same old place at the same old time, Dr. Merves-Okin says. Taking on different roles can make it seem like a new experience.

Look for new inspiration. High-quality erotic books and videos can show couples new ways to express their love. One such series comes from the Sinclair Intimacy Institute, which produces the *Better Sex Video Series* and *The Couples Guide to Great Sex over 40*. "These are very good educational films," says Dr. Whipple. But anytime you use erotica, both partners have to agree and be comfortable with it, she stresses.

Dress up for bed. Wearing a negligee or any other garment that seems sexy can make your love life feel a little more extraordinary. "It doesn't have to be a scanty nighty. It can be something that looks pretty and feels nice against your skin. Or maybe just wear a pretty robe. Whatever makes you feel sexy," Dr. Merves-Okin says.

may lead to the next step, but it doesn't have to." Dr. Whipple recommends trying to please each other without intercourse. Experiment and find other things that you enjoy—touching, kissing, cuddling.

Working with Your Changing Body

By the time we reach 50, our lives can be much more open to sexual pleasure. The kids are out of the house, we're more confident in ourselves, and we're not worried about getting pregnant. But our bodies are also going through changes that could get in the way of our sex life. "There are physical changes, but they aren't anything that can't be coped with," says Dr. Whipple.

The biggest change is in our estrogen levels, Dr. Whipple says. Although, on the average, we reach menopause in our early fifties, estrogen begins to decline as early as age 35. Low levels may cause vaginal dryness, which can make sex painful or uncomfortable. "Many women don't associate this problem with estrogen levels because at 35 they're not even thinking about those kinds of changes yet," she says. But left untreated, lack of lubrication can last through and past menopause.

These changes can be discouraging, but those who cope and adapt often find that their sex lives remain satisfying and may even get better than they have ever been. "You have to accept that change is inevitable in all aspects of our lives. What I liked at 25 isn't what I like at 40, but that doesn't mean what I liked at 25 was better. It doesn't mean your sex life is over. It just means it is different," Dr. Donahey says.

Here are some strategies to help you over the rough spots.

SEX SYMBOLS AT ANY AGE

Sex symbol: Two little words that evoke a gallery of images of beautiful and voluptuous young women.

Wait a minute. *Young?*

Plenty of women have shown us beyond a doubt that a woman can be sensuous and sexy at any age. Here's a short list, and there are lots more where they came from.

Mae West. At 43 years of age, Mae West was the highest paid woman in the United States, thanks mostly to the provocative, sometimes downright bawdy roles she played. At age 62, she starred in her own nightclub act (surrounded by muscle men). And in 1978, at the age of 85, she starred in the movie *Sextette*.

Eartha Kitt. Known for her smoldering, slinky performances, a 64-year-old Kitt played a seductress in the recent Eddie Murphy film *Boomerang*. Her 1992 memoir was titled *I'm Still Here: Confessions of a Sex Kitten*.

Raquel Welch. Renowned as much for her beauty and sexiness as for her acting, Welch, at age 57, was named one of the sexiest women in the world in a reader survey by *Shape* magazine and has played everything from bit parts to starring roles in films made both here and abroad. She's also made several exercise videos and has written two fitness books.

Sophia Loren. In her midsixties, the buxom Italian "goddess" is still considered a sex symbol by many and played the object of affection in the 1995 movie *Grumpier Old Men*.

Susan Sarandon. In a 1999 television movie, a 52-year-old Sarandon had an affair with a 25-year-old man. It wasn't the first time Sarandon showed how older women can be sensual and attractive to younger men. She was 13 years older than her love interest in *White Palace*, 12 years older than her boyfriend in *Thelma and Louise*, and 12 years older than her male counterpart in *Bull Durham* (actor Tim Robbins, with whom Sarandon has two children in real life).

Be open to change. For a premenopausal woman, it takes 6 to 20 seconds to lubricate after she is aroused. For a postmenopausal women, it takes 1 to 3 minutes. Instead of fearing these changes, work with them, Dr. Donahey says. You may have to take more time during sex, use sexual aids, or find other ways to please each other. Adapting to these changes can be fun and exciting, she says. Couples who have trouble during this time are often the ones who insist on doing everything the way they always have.

Apply a lubricant. Try some artificial lubrication to keep sex comfortable. Apply over-the-counter water-soluble lubricants (like K-Y jelly, Replens, or Astroglide) right before intercourse. Other products, such as Vagisil Intimate Moisturizer, can be used at any time. You can even make the application of a lubricant a pleasurable part of the sexual experience, Dr. Whipple says, instead of seeing it as something that reminds you of a problem.

Work out your pelvis. There's actually a workout for better sex. Kegel exercises strengthen the pelvic-floor muscles. To find your pelvic muscles, says Dr. Ladas, squeeze your pelvic area as if you were trying to stop the flow of urine. Once you've found them, squeeze, hold for 1 to 2 seconds, then relax. Repeat about 5 to 10 times at first. Try to work yourself up to squeezing and relaxing for 10 seconds each, 10 times in a row. She also suggests that you do what she calls "fast flicks": contract and relax those same pelvic muscles as rapidly as possible. Dr. Ladas recommends 100 of these a day.

Have sex as often as possible. Women who have sex two or more times a week have twice as much estrogen circulating in their blood as women who don't, Dr. Whipple says. By having more sex, you generate more estrogen, which lubricates the vagina, making sex easier for you.

Making the Most of Menopause

No more birth control! No more tampons or pads! No more premenstrual syndrome!

Once upon a time, we called it the change. It was a landmark that signaled the end of the best and most productive years of our lives. We avoided talking about it and tried not to think about it. But not anymore.

Most of the millions of women who will reach menopause over the next decade will still have a third of their lives ahead of them. As far as they're concerned, "the change" no longer means an end to anything. Instead, it heralds a new beginning.

Consider that in a recent Gallup poll of 750 women between the ages of 45 and 60, more than half viewed menopause as a fulfilling stage of life; 60 percent did not associate menopause with feeling less attractive; and a whopping 80 percent expressed relief over the end of menstruation.

"Culturally, we're beginning to look upon menopause as the start of a new life. You're free from your children and many other obligations. You can start a new career, go back to school, travel, open up a business. You are not going to be a hunched-over little old lady pushing a vol-unteer cart," says Mary Leong, M.D., director of gynecology at the Nassau County Medical Center in East Meadow, New York.

No one is pretending that *everything* about menopause is pleasant. All of the well-known side effects still happen to women, including hot flashes, mood swings, and vaginal dryness. But these days we can openly discuss these side effects and get far more information about how to deal with them.

Turning Down the Heat

It starts with a flush of warmth in your chest, then intensifies and quickly moves into your neck, face, and head. Your heart starts to beat faster and faster, and sweat forms on your skin as your body tries to cool off. As quickly as it comes, it can go but can last up to several minutes. It's a hot flash, and for many women, these sporadic moments of burning within are what menopause is all about.

"When you talk about symptoms, what actually causes women to come in to see a doctor are the hot flashes. It's the number one complaint about menopause," says Susan Johnson, M.D., professor of obstetrics and gynecology at the University of Iowa College of Medicine in Iowa City.

About 75 percent of women going through menopause experience hot flashes, although the intensity differs from woman to woman. Some women may only experience them for a month, while other women have them for 5 years.

While annoying, they pose no health risks. They're simply the sensation that comes along with changing hormonal balances in the body. "The only reason to treat hot flashes is if they bother you and you have trouble sleeping," Dr. Johnson says.

If you find the flashes unendurable, you can talk to your doctor about hormone-replacement therapy. But Dr. Johnson suggests that there's lots you can do to control your body's thermostat yourself.

Add soy to your diet. Soy contains phytoestrogens, natural substances that act very much like the estrogen your body makes. Some women find relief from hot flashes by eating soy-based foods such as soy milk or tofu. "There is pretty good evidence that soy provides relief, but it won't work for everybody," she says. Start with two 8-ounce glasses of soy milk a day. Once you get used to that, add tofu or other soy products to your diet. Don't expect immediate results. It can take from 6 to 8 weeks for you to feel its effects.

Take a deep breath. According to the North American Menopause Society, deep breathing can reduce hot flashes by 50 percent.

HRT: Should You or Shouldn't You?

When a woman enters menopause, her body begins to slow down its production of estrogen. That can cause problems ranging from hot flashes to osteoporosis. To relieve those symptoms, she can take hormones in the form of drugs, a treatment called hormone-replacement therapy, or HRT.

Some doctors prescribe HRT as commonly as they dispense aspirin. Yet others, such as Susan Johnson, M.D., professor of obstetrics and gynecology at the University of Iowa College of Medicine in Iowa City, aren't so sure that every woman going through menopause should be on it. "By and large, estrogen is safe, and it's a good solution for some women. But that doesn't mean everyone should be taking it," she says.

Before you decide whether hormone-replacement therapy is right for you, you'll need to know some facts. Here is what experts have learned from their research.

It solves symptoms. Short-term HRT helps alleviate menopausal symptoms such as hot flashes and vaginal dryness.

It's heart friendly. Long-term use of HRT may reduce the risk of heart disease. A major study found, however, that HRT did not reduce the risk of heart attacks in women who already had heart disease before taking HRT.

It makes bones stronger. Long-term use of HRT is the standard care for the prevention and treatment of osteoporosis.

It's risky for breasts. Long-term use is associated with increased risk of breast cancer.

In balance, it's a lifesaver. More women die every year of heart disease and osteoporosis-related conditions than breast cancer.

Take six to eight slow, deep abdominal breaths per minute. Practice for 15 minutes each morning and night, and breathe deeply when you feel a hot flash coming on.

Unfortunately, all the data doesn't point to an easy answer. Assuming that HRT will prevent heart disease and osteoporosis ignores other factors, such as diet, physical activity, obesity, and smoking, all of which contribute to the development of these diseases, Dr. Johnson says.

"If we have an overweight woman with diabetes and a strong family history of heart disease, then putting her on HRT makes sense," she adds. "But if we have a normal-weight, nondiabetic woman with normal cholesterol and whose family has no history of heart disease, then putting her on a preventive medication is ridiculous."

On the flip side, Dr. Johnson says that some women overestimate their breast cancer risk and shy away from HRT when it could help them prevent heart disease and osteoporosis.

Each woman, in conjunction with her doctor, must make up her own mind about hormone-replacement therapy. Consider these questions when deciding.

Long term or short term? There are two reasons to take HRT: for short-term relief of menopausal symptoms and for long-term prevention of heart disease and osteoporosis. Studies haven't shown any health risks associated with short-term (5 to 10 years) HRT, Dr. Johnson says. If you take it for disease prevention, however, you'll have to take it for the rest of your life.

What are your risks? Depending on a woman's individual health risks, HRT may or may not be a good choice. People at a higher-than-normal risk for heart disease and osteoporosis should consider HRT, while those at higher risk of breast cancer probably should not. Dr. Johnson recommends that you weigh your risk of each disease before making a decision.

Stay cool. Do your best to stay in cool areas during the day since heat or a dramatic temperature change can trigger a hot flash. During the summer, remain in air-conditioned rooms or use fans to keep your internal temperature from rising. During the winter, be careful not to turn the heater up too high.

Steer clear of triggers. For some women, certain foods or even situations can bring on a hot flash. Take note of what you ate or did right before a hot flash came on, so you can avoid it in the future. Caffeine, alcohol, and spicy foods are all common hot flash triggers.

Slumber in coolness. If you experience night sweats, turn the thermostat down or open a window when you go to bed. Make sure that the room is cool, yet comfortable. Wear light, comfortable night clothes and place a fan by your bed.

Go natural. Wear clothing made of natural fibers, such as cotton. Natural fibers allow heat and moisture to escape instead of trapping them against your skin.

Layer it on. Dress in layers, such as T-shirts under sweaters or long-sleeve shirts. Or wear vests and cardigans so that when a hot flash occurs, you can peel your clothes back off in layers to cool yourself down.

In the Mood

No one is quite sure how deep breathing works to help you. It may slow your metabolism, regulate your body temperature, or even control the brain chemicals associated with hot flashes.

Your body temperature isn't the only thing that can suddenly switch from one extreme to the other during menopause. You may also notice sudden mood changes. Some women report being very short-tempered and even somewhat depressed.

Even women who have experienced mood swings from premenstrual syndrome all their lives note that these are a bit more intense. "They find it is much more noticeable than it used to be," says Lisa Domagalski, M.D., a gynecologist and assistant clinical professor at Brown University School of Medicine in Providence, Rhode Island.

Experts aren't sure what links mood changes to menopause. It could be an estrogen connection, or it may have something to do with mood-altering brain chemicals, such as serotonin. Part of the difficulty may lie in sleep deprivation due to hot flashes and night sweats.

If your mood changes last a long time or impair your ability to work or function, or if you feel that you are slipping into a deep depression, see a doctor immediately. She will help you explore options such as medication and therapy. If your mood changes are causing you (and those around you) only minor grief, try the following strategies to get your emotions back on an even keel.

Walk or exercise often. In a study at Texas A&M University College of Medicine in College Station, women who walked 20 minutes reported significant improvements in mood. "Walking and exercise naturally increase the body's endorphins, chemicals in the body that make you feel good. That's where the 'high' that people get from running comes from," Dr. Domagalski says. People who exercise regularly have a much easier transition during menopause in general, she adds.

REAL-LIFE SCENARIO

What She's Not Doing to Protect Her Bones

At age 67, Anne's grandmother broke her hip. Afterward, tests showed she had osteoporosis. That fracture was only the first of many. At almost exactly the same age, Anne's mother fell and broke her shoulder. Same diagnosis. Now 49 and approaching menopause, Anne is determined to avoid the same fate by getting plenty of calcium and exercise. Each day she takes 600 milligrams of calcium carbonate first thing in the morning and last thing before bed. Since she skips breakfast, she makes sure to eat *real* (she hates the low-fat stuff) yogurt along with her salad at lunch. She loves cheese and eats it freely—heck, she has a great excuse! Though petite and only 110 pounds, she never gains weight, which she credits to her addiction to running and her abstinence from alcohol. Diet soda is her drink of choice, at least a six pack a day. Naturally, she was surprised to find out at her annual checkup last week that she's now 5 feet 3½ inches tall—½ inch shorter than she was a year ago. Should she be concerned?

Anne should be concerned. Her loss of height may be a symptom of bone loss. But she's already on the right track with her focus on weight-bearing exercise, calcium intake, and awareness of her risk. Some small mistakes in her daily routine, however, are subtracting the benefits of her bone-protecting strategies. With only a few changes, Anne should be able to preserve her bones, which would make her less likely to share her mother's and grandmother's fate.

First off, Anne should switch to calcium citrate. The calcium she takes, calcium carbonate, is the least absorbable type.

When buying her calcium citrate or any calcium product, Anne must check the back label for the number of mil-

Practice relaxing. In the early 1970s, Herbert Benson, M.D., at the Harvard Medical School devised the "relaxation response." This tension-releasing technique can help you ligrams of elemental calcium—the amount of pure calcium in each pill. For instance, there is only 20 percent of elemental calcium in each milligram of calcium carbonate. If the amount of elemental calcium or calcium is not given on the back label, when she takes 600 milligrams of calcium carbonate, she's really only getting 120 milligrams of calcium.

It's also important to take calcium supplements with meals. Calcium needs stomach acid to dissolve and be absorbed by your body. The only time you have stomach acid is when you eat. By taking calcium supplements without food, Anne is not absorbing any of it.

Anne should also space out her calcium intake better. You can't absorb more than 500 milligrams at a time. Anne should evenly divide her needed 1,200 to 1,500 milligrams over three meals, in either food or supplements. The best way to do so is to make sure that she eats calcium foods with every meal or at least take supplements. And by not eating breakfast, Anne is missing a great opportunity to get calcium at the start of her day.

Finally, Anne must cut back on her diet soda fixation. Soda contains caffeine and phosphoric acid, both of which cause the body to excrete calcium. At the least, Anne should cut back to only two cans of soda a day, perhaps substituting fat-free milk or calcium-fortified orange juice the rest of the time.

Expert consulted
Michael T. DiMuzio, Ph.D.
Assistant professor at Northwestern University
Evanston, Illinois
Director of the Osteoporosis Prevention and
    Research Centers at Highland Park Hospital
Highland Park, Illinois

ings of relaxation for you, perhaps a word like *calm* or *serene*. Repeat the word in your mind every time you exhale. Practice this for 20 minutes once a day or 10 minutes twice a day as well as anytime you feel your mood begin to change.

Reward yourself. If you're feeling down and blue, don't sit there and brood about it. Do something that makes you happy. Take a bubble bath, treat yourself to a massage, buy yourself a treat. With all that's going on in your life and your body, you deserve to nurture yourself, Dr. Johnson says.

Solving a Sexual Problem

Thanks to Mother Nature's birth control, your sex life can flourish after menopause. But there is one physical change that you'll have to overcome. The drop in estrogen that occurs during menopause may cause the lining of your vagina to thin. During this thinning process, the vagina can become shorter, narrower, and drier. For some women, these changes make sex unpleasant and even painful.

Vaginal dryness isn't a barrier to sex, but simply a physical change that you'll have to adapt to, says Beverly Whipple, R.N., Ph.D., professor of nursing at Rutgers College of Nursing in Newark, New Jersey, and president of the American Association of Sex Educators, Counselors, and Therapists. You may want to discuss hormone-replacement therapy with your doctor, but you have many avenues to keep your sex life sizzling during menopause and for years after.

through mood swings or periods of anxiety, Dr. Johnson says. Sit or lie down in a comfortable position and breathe deeply. Relax all your muscles. Think of a phrase or word that evokes feel-

PERI WHO? THE NEW KID ON THE BLOCK

We either have the cramps and mood swings of menstruation or the hot flashes and sleepless nights of menopause. Not much of a choice, is it? But guess what? There's actually a time when we can have all the symptoms at once!

It's called perimenopause.

The name itself means "near the end of menstruation." It's the time when your estrogen levels begin to decline, which triggers the symptoms of hot flashes, mood swings, and irregular periods, says Dori Becker, M.D., a physician at Highland Park Hospital in Highland Park, Illinois. While your body isn't producing as much estrogen as it did, it still produces some, so you still have all the symptoms associated with menstruation to deal with, too. Perimenopause lasts until you reach menopause, which happens when you have gone a full year without a period.

Perimenopause can start in your forties and can last up to 5 years, possibly even longer, Dr. Becker says. Because they're still getting periods, many women don't think of their symptoms as part of the process of menopause. Or they think they've reached early menopause. Both are misconceptions.

Women have always gone through perimenopause, of course. But giving it a name validates what a lot of women experience at this time of their lives. "I am really pleased that there is more press about this. My friends and patients are at this age and are noticing that things are beginning to change," says Wendy Fader, Ph.D., a licensed psychologist and certified sex therapist in Boca Raton, Florida.

Love to love. According to Dr. Whipple, having sex generates estrogen, even during menopause. Studies have shown that women who have sex two or more times a week maintain twice as much estrogen in their bodies as women who don't. As a "natural" estrogen-replacement therapy to help keep the vagina lubricated, continue to have sex regularly, either with a partner or by yourself, advises Dr. Whipple.

Use water-based lubricants. Over-the-counter lubricants make sex comfortable for both partners. When buying a lubricant, make sure that it is water-based like K-Y jelly, not oil-based, Dr. Whipple says. Oil-based lubricants take longer to dissolve and can make a comfortable breeding ground for germs. They can also cause latex-based products, such as condoms, to develop small holes and deteriorate.

Shake up your routine. You and your partner might have to get a bit more creative in the bedroom. You may need more foreplay before sex, or you might want to try other sexually pleasing acts that don't always include intercourse. Just like everything else in life, your sexual practices may need to change, and the people who do best are the ones who roll with the changes instead of fear them, says Karen Donahey, Ph.D., director of the sex and marital therapy program at Northwestern University Medical Center in Chicago.

Sweet Sleep
and Relaxation

Sleeping Beauty. Remember her story? She pricked her finger on a spindle, then slept for a hundred years.

Getting some rest should be so easy! In fact, women make up the majority of the 84 million Americans who experience insomnia at least occasionally, insomnia being the inability to get enough sleep.

How much is enough? According to Peter Hauri, Ph.D., codirector of the Sleep Disorders Center at the Mayo Clinic in Rochester, Minnesota, it varies from person to person. For some, as little as 4 hours will do, while for others, 9 hours is a must. The average person functions just fine on 7 to 8.

If you're not getting the sleep you need, you won't need to check into a rest home, but you may feel like you belong in one. It's probably no surprise that, among other things, sleep deprivation cuts energy levels, reduces your ability to concentrate, and can make you moody—affecting everything from your work performance and your relationships to your driving skills. Not to mention causing those other, yet all-important, eye "problems"—unsightly bags and circles.

On the other hand, getting the right amount of sleep can—overnight—help you to think, look, and feel younger. Just think what a little shut-eye did for Sleeping Beauty. When that handsome prince fell for her peaceful, resting face and woke her with a kiss, she was well over a hundred years old! Talk about a youth enhancer.

The Mind-Body Connection

So why is it so hard for some of us to crawl under the covers—and stay there? For one thing, sleep difficulties may be one of the consequences of leading an extremely busy life, says Meir Kryger, M.D., professor of medicine at the University of Manitoba in Winnipeg, Canada, and past president of the American Sleep Disorders Foundation. "In our society, we have demanding careers that extend beyond 5:00 P.M., extracurricular activities after we leave the office. We can watch 24-hour television, and we can stay up all night surfing the Internet," he explains.

But there are a variety of other factors, both

physical and psychological, says Martin Moore-Ede, M.D., Ph.D., chief executive officer of Circadean Technologies, a research and consulting firm in Cambridge, Massachusetts, that specializes in reducing workplace fatigue; a former professor of physiology at Harvard Medical School; and coauthor of *The Complete Idiot's Guide to Getting a Good Night's Sleep*. Here are some of the most common.

Illness. The quality of your sleep is a barometer of your health. Insomnia can result from depression or pain. It can also be caused by sleep apnea, a condition in which you stop breathing for 10 to 60 seconds at a time, then wake up for a few moments, then fall back asleep—sometimes without even being aware that your sleep has been disturbed. Restless leg syndrome, which makes your legs feel jumpy so that you have to move them to get relief, can also keep you awake. And then there's periodic limb movement disorder, which causes you to kick while sleeping. (The bruises on your partner's legs will tell you if you have this problem.)

External factors. Common lifestyle-related causes of sleep problems include drinking alcohol or caffeinated drinks late in the evening, eating foods that could cause heartburn before going to bed, arguing with your mate before bedtime, worrying about unfinished business from the workday, and engaging in vigorous exercise after 6:00 or 7:00 P.M. (Experts say that having sex is the exception to this rule; *that* type of exercise may actually help you release tension and relax.) An uncomfortable bed or a bed-

---

REAL-LIFE SCENARIO
She Doesn't Know How to Relax

At 40, Rosemary lives life to the fullest. She has a part-time job as a secretary with the local library. She cooks meals for her family, tries to exercise regularly, coordinates family activities, acts as a taxi service for her adolescent twins, and tries to maintain a happy marriage. On the weekends, she cleans house and does the laundry and grocery shopping. She's also on the building committee of her church, occasionally volunteers to distribute newspapers at the community hospital, and actively participates in an e-mail forum on environmental issues. Her one outlet for relaxation had been ballroom dancing, but she became so accomplished at it that she decided to teach and compete; thus her hobby has turned into a second job.

As engaged with her life as she feels, she's noticed lately that she's been experiencing headaches, and she's unable to sleep at night. In fact, sometimes she feels so old and tired and out of control of her life that she vacillates between losing interest in everything and frantically trying to keep up with it all, as if she's on the verge of a breakdown. What should she do?

Rosemary's life has become a merry-go-round, and she's at risk of falling off. She's an extrovert who has naturally gravitated toward people-oriented activities, but, unfortunately, she's overextended herself, and she's experiencing diminishing returns.

On the positive side, Rosemary has tried to create balance in her life by exercising, nurturing her family, and working no more than part-time. But she's a doer, and these types of people add more and more to their schedules until they wear themselves out, long before their time, both physically and psychologically. No wonder she's feeling old and tired.

---

rying about unfinished business from the workday, and engaging in vigorous exercise after 6:00 or 7:00 P.M. (Experts say that having sex is the exception to this rule; *that* type of exercise may actually help you release tension and relax.) An uncomfortable bed or a bed-

room that's too light, too hot, or too cold are also likely to stand between you and dreamtime.

Mind games. If you've been having trouble sleeping, you're more likely to begin worrying the moment you hit the sheets about whether

The solution is for her to adopt certain lifestyle changes that will help her comfortably ease out of her stressful situation and return to the youthful enthusiasm and energy she has a right to.

She should begin by setting aside an hour each day dedicated to herself: taking a bath, listening to music, or doing relaxation exercises such as rhythmic breathing, progressive relaxation (in which she tenses, then relaxes, one body part at a time), or autogenic training (which consists of self-suggestion relaxation techniques such as "My arms are feeling warm and heavy.").

Once she begins to let go of stress, she'll notice that she's feeling more alert, refreshed, and focused. From this calmer, more centered frame of mind, Rosemary should reflect on her life and priorities. Now she's in a position to simplify her life by focusing on the projects that are most important to her and letting go of the low-priority ones.

Realistically, given her personality type, Rosemary is still likely to keep herself busier than most women. To stay healthy, she'll need to incorporate relaxation exercises into her daily routine. For example, she should learn to recognize certain early warning signs of tension—such as tightening of the muscles in her jaw, neck, and shoulders—and use these internal cues as reminders to stretch, breathe deeply, and consciously release the stress.

Expert consulted
Martha Davis, Ph.D.
Author of The Relaxation and Stress
    Reduction Workbook
Psychologist
Department of psychology at Kaiser Perma-
    nente Medical Center
Santa Clara, California

asleep. This creates anxiety, which actually *does* prevent them from relaxing and falling asleep."

Turning Out the Lights, Naturally

Rest easy. There are lots of things that you can do to ensure a blissful night's sleep. Here are the very basic ones from the experts.

Make time. Allow yourself at least 45 minutes to an hour to unwind before you lie down in bed. Let the leftover tension from your long day drift away. Avoid working on finances or watching the late news or stimulating your mind in any way too close to bedtime.

Don't be a clock watcher. Remove your clock from your bedside; in fact, remove it from the room, if possible. A watched pot never boils, and a watched clock won't let you sleep.

Work it off early. Exercise regularly during the day and find as many waking outlets for your stress as possible. The object is to be physically and mentally stress-free by bedtime.

Cozy up. Create a comfortable bed and bedroom. From room temperature to the crispness of the sheets, everything should be just the way you like it when you turn in for the night.

you're going to have trouble sleeping again. It's a cruel irony of insomnia. "People learn behavior that prevents them from falling asleep," explains Dr. Kryger. "It's a conditioned reflex called psychophysiologic insomnia, in which people associate going to bed with having a problem falling

Easing toward Dreamland

It's no accident that children, whom one rarely hears complaining about sleeplessness, have an elaborate set of bedtime rituals. "Rituals are sequences of behavior that help you wind

WOMEN ASK WHY

Why do older people get up early when they don't have to?

Various stages of life bring changes in our sleep patterns. Aging appears to involve a resetting of our biological clocks, which causes us to experience the internal signals that tell us both when to wake up and when to go to sleep earlier in the day. This is most likely the result of changes in our bodies' release of melatonin, a hormone secreted by the pineal gland deep within the brain, which regulates the wake/sleep cycle.

Also, as you age, you're likely to notice that both the timing and the quality of your sleep are undergoing changes. For example, the older you get, the less time you'll spend in the deep stage 3 and stage 4 sleep, and the more (proportionately) you'll spend in stages 1 and 2—the lighter stages.

As a result of getting less satisfying sleep, you might find yourself becoming groggy and going to bed earlier in the evening. Because your body only requires a certain number of hours of sleep per night, you're likely to wake up earlier the following morning. That, in turn, may lead you to go to bed early that evening, and before you know it, you've established a new sleep pattern.

If this is the case and your internal clock is out of whack, reset it by going to bed 10 minutes later each night for 6 consecutive nights. Continue this regimen for several weeks, if necessary, until you are able to go to bed as late as you like. As for getting up early, relax and enjoy the time.

Expert consulted
Dian Dincin Buchman, Ph.D.
New York, NY
Author of The Complete Guide to Natural Sleep

Whatever comforting things you do before bed—throwing on your favorite pajamas, tucking in your sheets, or brushing your teeth—do them in the same order every night and take as many of them on the road with you as you can when you travel. Establishing and following a relaxation ritual that works for you is a key factor in avoiding sleep problems.

Here are some relaxing steps from experts that you might want to add to your bedtime ritual.

Sip a natural relaxer. Tranquilizing herbal tea blends made with chamomile (such as Celestial Seasonings Sleepytime Tea), valerian, or passionflower are age-old sleep aids for their ability to induce drowsiness, while warm milk contains tryptophan, a chemical that also helps make you sleepy, says Dr. Moore-Ede.

Create the mood. While getting into your before-bed mode, turn down the lights and illuminate with candles to create a soft, warm glow. While you're at it, choose candles with scented lavender, a fragrance known for its calming properties. (Just make sure to put out those candles before you finally turn in.)

Soothe your senses. Off with the car chases, bad sitcoms, and general blare of the TV, and on with soft music, a traditional relaxation tool. Choose jazz, classical, R&B—whatever style you prefer as long as it's smooth and mellow. Tuning in should help you tune out your troubles.

down and get ready for bed; it's part of the relaxation process," explains Dr. Moore-Ede. Even if you factor teddy bears and bedtime stories out of the equation, adults need bedtime rituals, too.

Engage your imagination. Reading poetry, short stories, or other relaxing fare can help transport your thoughts away from your world for a short time. Those who have a really hard time falling asleep should probably avoid thrillers, scary science fiction, and any other pulse-quickening genres.

Get that warm, fuzzy feeling. Since studies show that petting an animal can lower your blood pressure, bedtime might also be a good time to gently brush your dog or cuddle your cat—in turn, treating yourself to a bit of furry relaxation therapy.

Immerse yourself. Slipping into a warm bath for 20 minutes can ease the transition from a stressful day to a quiet evening. As the heat helps open blood vessels and relaxes tired muscles, let your mind drift to pleasant thoughts, says Dr. Kryger.

Calm your mind. Prayer and meditation can also bring peace and allow you to shut off the cares of the day. They require some self-discipline and may take a little practice, but it's time well spent a few minutes before bed.

Tap the power of touch. If you're fortunate enough to have a partner with you, exchange light, not-too-stimulating massages. If you're alone, you can still gently run your hands over your own body, feeling yourself relax as you go along.

Get into a rhythm. Practicing rhythmic breathing can help take your focus off your mind and direct it toward your body. Simply breathe deeply—filling first your stomach and then your lungs with air—and exhale slowly, allowing yourself to become more drowsy and calm each time you exhale.

Stretch your limits. Stretching or tensing muscles one at a time for a few seconds and then relaxing them helps release tension. And a relaxed body is one that will drift off to sleep easily, says Dr. Kryger.

When All Else Fails

What if you still can't fall asleep? Should you take medication?

"Sleeping pills and tranquilizers can be helpful in the short term," says Dr. Hauri. "They allow you to get to sleep if you're in a different time zone and absolutely need to be well-rested and alert, or if there's been a death in the family, and the grief and stress have made it impossible for you to sleep. But if you're taking them more than once or twice a week, that may be a problem. Anytime your inability to sleep interferes seriously with your daytime functioning for more than a month or two, that's the time to seek professional help," he says.

Indeed, if your insomnia is chronic, says Dr. Moore-Ede, "you should try to work your way around medication; you're far better off dealing with the environmental and lifestyle issues that are likely to be keeping you awake."

Index

Underscored references indicate boxed text. **Boldface** page references indicate illustrations.